MY
Sleep
AND *I*

TERESA PAIVA

Copyright © 2024 by Teresa Paiva

Paperback: 978-1-964744-87-2
eBook: 978-1-964744-88-9
Library of Congress Control Number: 2024916396

Ordering Information:

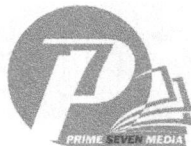

Prime Seven Media
518 Landmann St.
Tomah City, WI 54660

Printed in the United States of America

Reasons for reading this book

This book is organised in chapters aiming to provide a personalised view of normal and abnormal sleep.

The first section – My Sleep – provides a small theoretical review of the functions of sleep, explaining why we should sleep

The other sections talk about normal sleep, bad sleep, good and bad habits, sleep risks and stories around sleep disorders. Each chapter is a small history collected in real life, which is followed by a simple scientific explanation, with international references.

The main aim is to allow the recognition of your own possible problems so that you achieve better sleep and better quality of life.

So:

If you go late to bed
If we sent messages throughout the night
If you play with your PlayStation and/or work with your pc until quite late
If you are sleepless before your tests, exams or conferences
If you go to the disco and come home after sun rise
If you are sleepy because you curtail your sleep
If you wake up tired
If you wake up with a dull headache
If nobody and nothing can wake you up
If you wake with the noise of a fly
If you suffer from insomnia and don't sleep well
If you snore or stop breathing
If you don't have a restorative sleep
If you fall asleep anywhere
If strange things occur while you sleep
If you are more tired upon awakening than at sleep onset
If you are unable to follow regular schedules

If you are dissatisfied with your sleep
If you have strange or unpleasant dreams
If you dream across the night and wake up exhausted
If you sleep well but would like to know why
                              Then,

                                        This book is for you

A secondary didactic aim also exits

So:

If you want to understand
        How sleep matters in your daily life
        How sleep matters for your health
        How sleep matters for your survival
        How sleep matters for your success
        How sleep matters for your quality of life
        Why your sleep is not good
        Which are the risks of sleep curtailing
        Which disorder you likely have
        Which are the risks of a poor sleep
        Which are the consequences of sleeping too much
        How habits interfere with your health and your sleep
Then,

                                        This book is for you

A tertiary aim exists

So:

If you are a beginner in sleep medicine
        Want to understand patients' complaints in their own words
        Need to have simple bibliographic reviews of each theme
If you are a professional needing fast and simple updates
Then,

                                        This book is for you

Contents

A. My Sleep

1. WHY SLEEP?

We sleep to assure our survival, our physical health, our mental health, adequate performance in whatever field, quality of life and wellbeing, and a long and happy life

a) Survival

Survival is a fundamental and universal feature of living beings. Sleep appeared millions of years ago in pluricellular animals and persisted through evolution, despite the danger of exposure to predators. Sleep achievements were biologically superior when compared to the predation danger, since they assured survival. Interspecies transmission of sleep was quite successful, and, in that way, sleep exists in all animals so far studied.

In humans sleep survival is assured since foetal life, the preborn baby dreams most of the time, in his dreams he is learning the behaviours which will assure survival upon birth: crying in a way that someone will take care of him, rooting (infant's tendency to turn their head towards a touch stimulus, which facilitates nipple approach), sucking for feeding (babies adjust sucking pressure based on the flow of milk by sensing the upcoming flow), head turning (ability to lift and turn head to keep airway clear)[1] and motor protection by the Moro reflex[2].

---

[1] https://www.physiopedia.com/Understanding_Newborn_Behaviour#:~:text=The%20newborn%20has%20three%20survival,and%20events%20in%20the%20environment.

[2] Edwards CW, Al Khalili Y. Moro Reflex. [Updated 2023 Jul 25]. In: StatPearls [Internet]. Treasure Island (FL): StatPearls Publishing; 2024 Jan-. Available from: https://www.ncbi.nlm.nih.gov/books/NBK542173/

In adult life besides the positive sleep functions upon cognition, decision making, performance and health which are essential for survival, dreams of the sleeping brain are fundamental survival tools, since they allow behaviour training without danger.

Furthermore, during sleep brain monitors the environment, microarousals keep the brain and body prepared for any eventuality, and arousal threshold shows a marked duality, it is high for non-relevant stimuli, and low for relevant ones: we will wake when the baby cries or someone tries to open the door.

b) **Physical health**

Sleep is together, with nutrition and physical activity, a fundamental pillar of HEALTH[3]

Risks to our body related to bad sleep or sleep deprivation are numerous.

Why?

During sleep periods, anabolic hormones (the growth hormone, prolactin and testosterone) are systematically and regularly produced, and the catabolizing hormones are regulated, particularly cortisol and the thyroid stimulating hormone, which increase in case of sleep deprivation.

It all happens in a way that, while you sleep, you grow or repair tissues in different organs while reproductive functions and cell division are regulated. In the morning while waking up, cortisol is at an adequate level, for the day to start well. But if you do not get enough sleep,

---

[3] Knutson KL. Associations between sleep, diet, and exercise: implications for health and well-being.In: Foundations of Sleep Health, Eds F.Javier Nieto, Donna J. Petersen, Academic Press, 2022, Chapter 6,Pages 123-131, ISBN 9780128155011, https://doi.org/10.1016/B978-0-12-815501-1.00013-2.

anabolic hormones diminish and catabolizing hormones increase, and health risks start to appear.

Sleep has a "core" need. It should not be neither "too short" nor "too long". Health risks occur in the extremes of sleep duration[4,5].

Hypertension, cardiovascular and cerebrovascular problems appear with increased risks. Sleep duration between 6-8h has the lowest risk of cardiovascular events[6].

Furthermore, growth impairment can occur in children, while in adults the impact is upon tissue repair: wrinkles and weaker bones may become a problem.

On the other hand, sleep is essential in energy regulation and in homeostasis, for temperature control, which goes down while we sleep, and for energy control through feeding, in a balance that diminishes our hunger, if you sleep, or increases it in case of sleeplessness. For all this, having not enough sleep leads to fatigue, increases weight gain risk in all age groups, namely young children, together with the increased prevalence of type 2 diabetes.

Sleep has also a narrow and complex relation with immunity, and not sleeping increases the chance for infectious diseases and eventually auto-immune diseases.

[4]   Itani O, Jike M, Watanabe N, Kaneita Y. Short sleep duration and health outcomes: a systematic review, meta-analysis, and meta-regression. Sleep Med. 2017 Apr;32:246-256. doi: 10.1016/j.sleep.2016.08.006. Epub 2016 Aug 26. PMID: 27743803.

[5]   Jike M, Itani O, Watanabe N, Buysse DJ, Kaneita Y. Long sleep duration and health outcomes: A systematic review, meta-analysis and meta-regression. Sleep Med Rev. 2018 Jun;39:25-36. doi: 10.1016/j.smrv.2017.06.011. Epub 2017 Jul 5. PMID: 28890167.

[6]   Wang C, Bangdiwala SI, Rangarajan S, Lear SA, AlHabib KF, Mohan V, Teo K, Poirier P, Tse LA, Liu Z, Rosengren A, Kumar R, Lopez-Jaramillo P, Yusoff K, Monsef N, Krishnapillai V, Ismail N, Seron P, Dans AL, Kruger L, Yeates K, Leach L, Yusuf R, Orlandini A, Wolyniec M, Bahonar A, Mohan I, Khatib R, Temizhan A, Li W, Yusuf S. Association of estimated sleep duration and naps with mortality and cardiovascular events: a study of 116 632 people from 21 countries. Eur Heart J. 2019 May 21;40(20):1620-1629. doi: 10.1093/eurheartj/ehy695. PMID: 30517670; PMCID: PMC6528160.

While asleep, cell division is controlled, therefore short sleep, out of hours sleep or irregular sleep increase the chance of cancer in both genders.

Sleep deprivation also has behavioural consequences such as higher chance of trauma, unintentional accidents in children, adolescents and adults.

Good sleep, Good Health!

Synthesis: the risks and consequences of poor sleep for physical health are terrible. In all ages and in all continents, not enough sleep or too much sleep, increase the risk of obesity, hypertension, type II diabetes, accidents, cancer, cardio/cerebro vascular and autoimmune diseases

c) Mental Health and Cognition

Sleep is essential for learning, memory, decision making, creativity and emotional balance.

Sleep disturbances impact emotions, cognition and mental health

Why?

Because during sleep, our brain, released from the focus given to the external world, shifts and focus on itself and towards our body; and both these dialogues are essential to our health.

During Sleep, the old paradigm "a sound mind in a sound body" reaches its maximum intensity.

Our brain takes care of itself, increasing the intensity of sleep in more stimulated areas while awake, reconnecting important circuits and bonding quick interconnections between cerebral zones that speak with one another, while disconnecting unnecessary circuits to rest, and deleting irrelevant information while strengthening those which matters, i.e., a clean-up function of not useful information and toxic metabolites.

Since one does not learn what one does not like, a sleeping brain stabilizes emotions; since, in order to learn one must try, our brain creates, through dreams, virtual realities where, without risk, one can argue, run, fight, talk or cry, in a safe learning environment. Innovative dreams are about the impossible or the never seen, fostering the creativity required for creative work and for survival.

In teenagers and children, loss of sleep increases distractibility and irritability, in opposition to adequate sleep, which consolidates memory. In these ages risk behaviours, such as violence and fights, drugs, early sex, excessive screen time and sedentarism increase with sleep deprivation.

On the other hand, sleep deprivation affects memory of neutral and positive stimuli. This effect leads to remembering negative stimuli, and enhances behavioural tendencies towards impulsiveness and negative feelings, and, to a lower expression of emotional stimuli.

The connection between Sleep and Intellect has been indirectly appraised through correlations between some sleep characteristics, namely sleep spindles, and the IQ (Intelligence Quotient).

It is known that a sleep episode following a learning period will enhance what was previously learned. This is said to be true for verbal tasks, motor tasks, special orientation tasks and more specialized performances, such as playing music.

On the other hand, the daytime apprenticeship of a motor task is related and linearly correlated with the increase of delta activity and sleep spindles, in the following sleeping period, in the contralateral motor region.

The effects of sleep upon memory consolidation have been described in early 19th and 20th century, but there is presently a significant number of papers on the matter, restating this sleep function. On the other hand, sleep enhances and protects declarative memory.

It is known since the 1960's that declarative memory is affected by sleep or by sleep deprivation. A 36h sleep deprivation significantly diminishes the temporal sequence retention, even if aided by heavy doses of caffeine, and affects the correct perception of our own performance.

The idea that sleep enhances creativity was put forward by reports concerning several scientists and artists who have reported that creation of their masterpieces occurred right after waking up, after a dream or during a hypnagogic state.

A more detailed disclosure is due to Kekulé, concerning a dream that led him to the discovery of the benzene ring. Others can be also mentioned: The discovery of the sewing machine gearings, Dali's paintings, Mr. Jeckyll's Book by Stevenson, Paul McCartney's Imagine, Kurosawa's "Dreams" film, amongst many others.

The effect of sleep is not only to code and consolidate memories or learning, but rather to integrate them into new associative schemes, that through generalization or integration, could show new perspectives or directions, giving reason to the popular saying: "The pillow brings good advice".

Several experiments were conducted towards proving this integration capacity "again", in adults as well as in pre-lingual children.

In summary, nocturnal sleep allows, for all age groups, the consolidation of memories, and enhances concepts of information generalization, and the identification of hidden solutions.

Knowledge concerning the effects of sleep on emotions comes from the increase in irritability and bad temper after a sleep deprivation night, characteristics that worsen if sleep deprivation is repeated. Nonetheless, it is also known that acute deprivation can also have an antidepressant effect, used for years ago in the treatment of serious depressions.

On the other hand, it is known that both stress and positive or negative emotions happening during the day affect sleep.

An increase in positive events contributes to a better subjective sleep, and a good night's sleep enhances the recognition of images with positive emotional components. Negative events worsen sleep to many people, either good or bad sleepers.

In this perspective, sleep deprivation functions both as a bomb for irritability outbreaks in normal life and may explain depressive humour in many psychiatric disturbances.

Thus, the habit of sleeping less in intellectual workers of many working fields, from universities to finances and politics, significantly affects reasoning capabilities (memory, learning, creativity), executive functions and emotional abilities, which are essential to the execution of the intellectual tasks at hand.

To think right, it's important to sleep right!

Synthesis: Depression, insomnia and risk behaviours in all ages, burnout, dementia, some neurologic and psychiatric diseases are not only increasing in prevalence, but also revealing their high societal costs. Their relationship with sleep is clear.

d) Wellbeing, happiness, longevity

Health-related quality of life (HRQOL) is an individual's or a group's perceived physical and mental health over time. It is a multi-dimensional concept that includes domains related to physical, mental, emotional, and social functioning. Studies evaluating HRQOL in relation to sleep duration in large epidemiologic studies in adults[7] and

---

[7] Reis C, Dias S, Rodrigues AM, Sousa RD, Gregório MJ, Branco J, Canhão H, Paiva T. Sleep duration, lifestyles and chronic diseases: a cross-sectional population-based study. Sleep Sci. 2018 Jul-Aug;11(4):217-230. doi:10.5935/1984-0063.20180036. PubMed PMID: 30746039; PubMed Central PMCID: PMC6361301.

adolescents[8] and in sleep disorders Insomnia, narcolepsy[9], proved the deleterious effect of sleep reduction and sleep dysfunction upon HRQOL.

Both short and long sleep duration are associated with a greater risk of premature death[10].

One aspect of life fulfilment deals with successful ageing and longevity. The relationship between happiness and longevity has been studied in USA: the risk of death over the follow-up period is 6% among individuals who are "pretty happy" and 14% higher among those who are "not happy", independently of marital status, socioeconomic status, census division, and religious attendance[11].

Sleep well, Live longer!

Synthesis: The relationship between sleep and health related quality of life, happiness and longevity is clear.

[8]   Matos MG, Marques A, Gaspar T, Paiva T Perception of quantity and quality of sleep and their association with healthrelated quality of life and life satisfaction during adolescence. Health Edu Care, 2017 2(2): 1-6. ISSN: 2398-8517

[9]   David A, Constantino F, Santos JM, Paiva T. Health-related quality of life in Portuguese patients with narcolepsy. Sleep Med. 2012 Jan 24. [Epub ahead of print] PubMed PMID: 22281002.

[10] Cappuccio FP, D'Elia L, Strazzullo P, Miller MA. Sleep duration and all-cause mortality: a systematic review and meta-analysis of prospective studies. Sleep. 2010 May;33(5):585-92. doi: 10.1093/sleep/33.5.585. PMID: 20469800; PMCID: PMC2864873.

[11] Lawrence EM, Rogers RG, Wadsworth T. Happiness and longevity in the United States. Soc Sci Med. 2015 Nov;145:115-9. doi: 10.1016/j.socscimed.2015.09.020. Epub 2015 Sep 18. PMID: 26421947; PMCID: PMC4724393

2. HOW ARE SOCIETIES INFLUENCING SLEEP?

With the discovery of electricity, industrial and technological development allowing control over energy, food production, telecommunications, internet, artificial Intelligence, spatial industry, the social paradigms changed.

"To have", "To win", "Success", "No limits" become mandatory rules.

With globalization international societies changed and developed new habits and new work modalities.

Society is now continuously "on", first 24h per day, and then 7 days per week. Enjoyments changed and extended through the night. In this setting, Sleep became an embarrassment for work, productivity, amusement and economic interests.

Therefore, since last century, people have been sleeping less and less, and this deficit extends to all age categories.

The El Dorado of progress has however its black sides: The number of poor is increasing, and millions are beneath the poverty threshold; divorce and single parent families increase; wars and social instabilities emerge in several continents; uncertainty must be taken seriously; knowledge and erroneous myths circle freely on the internet; the climate crisis is in progression.

Sleep deprivation and related illnesses are serious issues. Societal economic costs related to sleep deprivation in the richest world countries are huge: $680 Billion are lost each year across five OECD countries (USA, Canada, UK, Japan, Germany) due to insufficient sleep[12].

---

[12] Hafner M, Stepanek M, Taylor J, Troxel WM, van Stolk C. Why Sleep Matters-The Economic Costs of Insufficient Sleep: A Cross-Country Comparative Analysis. Rand Health Q. 2017 Jan 1;6(4):11. PMID: 28983434; PMCID: PMC5627640.

The warnings about the risks of this sleeplessness are many, but in the global society they do not speak loud enough, choked by the systematic challenges and incentives in the opposite direction.

Sleeplessness is quite expensive!

Synthesis: Citizens must protect themselves against the 24/7 society, trying to take most of the benefits and the least of pain

In the following stories YOU are the MAIN THEME and the TARGET AUDIENCE

B. Sleep biodiversity

Humans are ecosystems, either individually or as groups (family, city, country etc).

"A sustainable ecosystem is one that, over the normal cycle of disturbance events, maintains its characteristic diversity of major functional groups, productivity, and rates of biogeochemical cycling"[13].

Sustainable ecosystems have a marked biodiversity. Biodiversity is patent inter genders, inter ages, inter individuals, inter countries, inter regions, inter races, etc.

Biodiversity is essential for humans and its reduction is considered among the possible causes of extinction. It is, in fact, one of the possible explanations of Neanderthals' extinction

So, let's be different!

Sleep follows this biodiversity; there are marked interindividual differences in the multiple sleep features.

Sleep characteristics and parameters are usually distributed in the population with a gaussian distribution, i.e. a distribution with a bell shape, the most common are at the dome of the bell, the least common at the outer borders.

---

[13]   Principles of Ecosystem Sustainability https://www.journals.uchicago.edu/doi/epdf/10.1086/285969

1. I LOVE SLEEPING

I love sleeping.

I have my little routines before sleeping. After taking off my make-up, I brush my teeth and so on, go to bed, read a little - I always have a book to read at night – and after reading a few pages I turn off the light.

In bed I like to feel the sheets against my skin and stretching my body so I can get into a comfortable position to sleep. I like to stretch and yawn.

It's what cats do, stretching out in enjoyment, their muscles taut with obvious pleasure.

I switch off the light and do not even realise I am falling asleep.

I am certainly not one to count sheep. I think I do not think about anything and if I do think, I do not notice it.

I love my bed. Waking up in the night? No way! Just one long period of sleep and I almost never dream. That is, I rarely dream. When I have slept a few hours longer I dream of something. Pleasant dreams!

I do not recall any insomnia. I do not remember having nightmares. I can sleep in any bed, and noise does not particularly worry me. I cannot sleep sitting down and I cannot sleep when my feet are cold, but in winter I put on some woollen socks and there you go... and on aeroplanes I know I don't sleep well (I am always envious of those who travel executive class).

I sleep peacefully and I do not mess up the bed. I don't dream often, and I quickly forget my dreams. Nothing special has ever happened to me during my sleep, except occasionally talking when I am more tired than normal. I say vague things, then. My husband once told me that I categorically stated that: "The elephants are all mine" and that he managed to have a conversation with me. When I woke up,

I had no recollection, nor had any idea of which elephants I was referring to.

If I wake up early, before 8 o'clock, and if I am tired, a little afternoon nap is wonderful. I lie down… I in the bed … the sofa will not do. I close the window, make the room dark and I am asleep. I wake up fresher than a daisy, ready for any work.

When I wake up in the morning, I feel good, smiling at the new day. In case I have to set my alarm clock or wake up too early, awakening is not so easy.

I hate my alarm clock and if I wake up before the right time, it is a drag, as I go out of bed without knowing what I am doing or what I want to do, I drop things, bump into bed and spill my coffee.

I need 8 or 9 hours to be fine, and everything seems fine.

Sleep is one of the pleasures of my life.

Sleep is my Superpower!

The act of sleeping is shared by countless animal species and has been vital to their survival for billions of years.

Those who sleep well fall asleep quickly, do not remember waking up, though they have tiny waking up instances during the night, and do not remember dreaming, though they have done so, and wake up in a good mood[14].

Those who sleep well have a great capacity to adapt to adverse conditions, stress, things which disturb sleep, etc.

Falling asleep involves certain rituals which we humans also share with animals: Dogs go round and round before lying down to

---

14   InformedHealth.org [Internet]. Cologne, Germany: Institute for Quality and Efficiency in Health Care (IQWiG); 2006-. In brief: What is "normal" sleep? [Updated 2022 Mar 14]. Available from: https://www.ncbi.nlm.nih.gov/books/NBK279322/

sleep, cats prepare their bed and purr, birds strike their nocturnal pose and organise themselves in their own complex manner, etc.

Sleeping implies assuming a position. For us sleeping lying down and sleeping in a bed is better than sleeping sitting down. Just like us, animals have their own sleeping postures.

Finally, to fall and to remain asleep a suitable temperature is needed. You cannot sleep when it is cold or too hot, if your feet are cold or very hot. The temperature around our face, or the snout of animals, is a universal constant at the moment of falling asleep, which is equal for all latitudes, and for hot and cold climates. This is why we tend to cover the face (or snout) when it is cold and uncover it when it is hot.

Falling asleep is quite characteristic. Prior one starts blinking and then nodding. The brain oscillates between slow and fast rhythms, the eye movements are slow and drifting, waking up is easy. The muscles relax but some brisk movements are possible, with falling down sensation, the thoughts are drifting, reaction time slows down.

During sleep we change position several times and go through several sleep cycles which last approximately 90 minutes in adults. In each cycle we figuratively "go up and down", that is, after falling asleep we move through light sleep to deep sleep, then light sleep again followed by REM sleep and a temporary awakening. This sequence of stages is well organized and repeats itself around 4 to 6 times a night. There are, however, things which can happen in each one of the stages and in the transition between them.

In deep sleep, also called stage N3[15] or slow wave sleep, the brain is very slow, cardiac and respiratory rhythms go down, it is very

---

[15] According to the new sleep classification deep sleep has a single stage called stage N3. In older literature it was made up of stages 3 and 4 or slow wave sleep. See The AASM Manual for the Scoring of Sleep and Associated Events https://aasm.org/clinical-resources/scoring-manual/

difficult to wake up and hormones are produced, such as the growth hormone. Body and brain temperature drop significantly. Dreams are rare and limited to abstract thoughts with extremely reduced memories. This sleep is essential and if we are sleep deprived it will be the first to be compensated for, since certain essential functions are carried out, namely those dealing with "homeostasis", or the internal equilibrium of our organism. It is also here that the body recovers from the wears and tears of wakefulness. When deprived of slow wave sleep we find it difficult to carry out our tasks and become "groggy" with impaired discernment. If we suddenly wake from this stage, we cannot recompose ourselves and we may become temporarily confused. Sleepwalking, night terrors and confusional arousals take place at the end of this period, when the transition to waking up is abnormal. This stage, which predominates in the first half of sleep, takes up around 20% of the whole night in an adult; it is more prolonged in children, but reduces with age.

In light sleep, made up of stages 1 and 2, the brain is moderately slow and sometimes a little unstable. Small bursts of fast brain activity occur which protect the cerebral cortex from waking up; they are called sleep spindles. There is some reactivity to external stimuli and our cortex reacts to them with some typical elements, called K-complexes or vertex sharp waves. The ability to wake up is moderate. This stage occupies around 50% of the night. Dreams are possible but not very common with limited recollection. In N2 multiple normal and abnormal phenomena occur. Talking in your sleep (called somniloquy) is relatively normal if not excessive but shouting or making another type of noise (snoring, grunting, etc.) is abnormal. Sleep apnoea (breathing arrest), enuresis (bed-wetting), myoclonus (brief twitching of limbs) and many other phenomena mainly occur during this stage.

In REM sleep the brain becomes relatively swift once more, with rapid eye movements, as if being pulled from one side to another, the heart speeds up and slows down, breathing is irregular, body temperature is no longer regulated and therefore subject to the temperature in the room, muscles are paralysed, and we dream. Spontaneous waking is frequent, but it is difficult to wake somebody up in REM sleep. The most fully developed dreams occur during this sleep stage, which predominates in the second half of the night by taking up around 20% of the total sleep time in an adult. There is a greater recollection of dreams. Newborn babies spend between 60% to 80% of total sleep time in REM. It was in fact through observing the sleep of his baby son that Kleitman realised that rapid eye movements existed, and he suggested studying them to Aserinsky. Both described REM sleep in 1953. REM stands for Rapid Eye Movement. Michel Jouvet, a French researcher, one of the pioneers in the study of REM sleep, called it paradoxical, due to the disparities in apparently strange things which happen in this stage, and the difficulty of understanding the usefulness that many disconnected events provide. It is also an essential stage, and following sleep deprivation, our body tries to compensate for lost REM sleep. It has key functions in learning, memory organization and psycho-affective stability. It is during this stage that cardio-circulatory problems may occur in susceptible individuals. It is also here that nightmares and REM parasomnias (RBD – REM Behaviour Disorder) occur.

Sleep represents a partial disconnection from the outside world, which despite the associated survival risks, has been maintained and developed to introduce other obvious advantages. However, during sleep in fact we are not totally isolated from the outside world, since we continue to monitor, even if in a slower manner, what is taking place through our senses of hearing and feelings.

The somatic sensory system warns us of cold, pain or other internal or external discomforts. We no longer see the external world, but our dreams produce our own private cinema.

During sleep several functions are carried out, such as:

- *All the anabolic hormones, in particular the growth hormone, prolactin and testosterone, are segregated. The growth hormone is produced during the first sleep cycle. As such, sleep is essential for everybody and particularly children, and the popular saying "Sleep makes you grow" is true.*
- *The production of "catabolic" hormones, such as cortisol, is controlled. When you curtail your sleep, cortisol is higher in the morning increasing hypertension risk.*
- *The metabolism is controlled, namely for carbohydrates and lipids. Chronic sleep deprivation increases the risk of type 2 diabetes and obesity in all age groups.*
- *Immunological processes are stabilized, namely the body's resistance to infections. A reduction in sleep increases the probability of contracting infectious diseases.*
- *Sleep has important controls over cell division mechanisms, and both chronic sleep deprivation and chronic hypnotic consumption increase the risk of cancer.*
- *The brain and body temperature and metabolism in general are reduced. Therefore, when we sleep we have to cover ourselves; otherwise we would wake up cold.*
- *Various cognitive functions, mainly those to do with memory, problem solving, creativity and learning, are established and rooted.*
- *Dreams enable emotional equilibrium to be restored and allow rehearsal of our problems and danger in a safe virtual environment.*
- *Besides all of this, one of the main functions of sleep is to keep us awake. If we do not sleep enough, we are sleepy, unable to carry out our daily tasks, while having an increased accident risk.*

Make your sleep a good thing in your life. Don't mistreat it! Sleep is a blessing!

2. STRONG, FRAGILE AND NORMAL SLEEPERS

Rita: I am sorry I am late, but I find it difficult getting up early.

John: We noticed! I can handle anything: going to bed late, going to bed early, not sleeping, sleeping just a little or quite a lot. Whatever the case, I sleep, and everything is always OK! I just need 8 hours to be fine.

Paula: How horrible. Not me! I must be careful. I always go to bed at the same time. If I go to bed later, I ruin everything. I do fall asleep, but I wake up shortly afterwards.

John: When I work through the night - occasionally before a conference or something like that, in the morning I feel fine – the lack of sleep only hits me later, but I hold on during the day and sleep fine at night.

Paula: I must be very careful. There are a lot of things that disturb my sleep: light, noise... I have to be in darkness and in silence. Any noise awakes me up.

Laura: I need to sleep 7 to 7 and half hours. I sleep a bit more at the weekend, but I don't like to stay in bed for hours...

John: Not me, nothing can wake me up – train, thunder, phone... and at the weekend I sleep even more. My wife gets annoyed since she must deal with the kids when they are up at 7 or 8 o'clock in the morning dancing and running around the house.

Paula: You are lucky! My child also wakes me up early so I can't catch up at the weekend. But even if I could, I wouldn't because if I oversleep, I get an headache.

Maggie: My husband is like you. He sleeps soundly. He likes to sleep with the window open and, I cannot stand neither the cold nor the light. We do not adjust very well about sleeping. I like to watch TV in bed and sleep late. He likes to go to bed early. I like sleeping with the cat, he hates cats and closes the door so the cat cannot come in. He gets up early as bright as a daisy — he looks after the kids — and I am only really functioning and awake halfway through the morning.

Laura: I hope this is the only thing you don't see eye to eye about...

Maggie: Very funny... but the truth about what you are thinking is that we also have different daily rhythms - he is a morning person, and I am so sleepy then, I am a night owl and he is then so sleepy, ... but, with care, we can get some good moments together.

Richard: Me and Gaby are not like that at all. We both sleep and with equal schedules. I have always slept well — around 7 hours except when my dad died. Then I went through some tough nights — when he got sick, and when he passed away, I didn't sleep for some time, up all night thinking... but after some time I got back to sleeping well.

Laura: Me too. When I am worried, I sleep worse, but when I sleep really well is when I go to my judo classes. Sleep is then strong and sound.

Richard: That happened to me too.

Joanna: Nothing like that for me. I need to sleep 9 or 10 hours. I have even had up to 20 hours on the trot, and I often sleep 14 hours at the weekend, because during the week I haven't been able to get enough sleep since I came to work here.

John: Wow, look at Joanna, she can talk! I thought she was in the clouds, but she's down here after all!

Bob: Did you see that guy on TV? He sleeps 5 hours a night, goes jogging in the morning, and never stops! I am just like him as well. Give me five hours sleep and I wake up happy as a lark.

Joanna: Don't take it as a sign of intelligence; the other day I heard that some brainy person slept a lot. Sounds just like me.

Rita: Yeah, I have also heard that waking early doesn't make your head swell. I wonder who invented the phrase "early to bed, early to rise?"

John: Well, it certainly wasn't you, and I am sure you wouldn't recommend it.

Bob: I'd like to chat more, but I must go and work.

Laura: There goes the worker...

Jayne: Let him go. But I am going to tell you something funny anyway: There's a friend of mine who sleeps with 7 cats; when I heard that my mouth fell open, because I cannot take any weight on top of me, blankets, clothes, whatever.

Rita: How horrible! Must be worse than sleeping with a husband who snores!

Joanna: Well, my dog sleeps on the floor by the bed, and even so he sometimes snores and wakes me.

Paula: I don't think it's a good idea to sleep with animals. It must be just like having a crying baby which doesn't let you fall asleep.

Maggie: You are right. I have started sleeping much worse since I had Michael. I think it's always like that. I used to drink an expresso at the end of dinner, but now I can't: a white night follows. I still smoke my peaceful cigarette before lying down.

Jayne: Peaceful cigarette?!

Maggie: Yes, when everybody else is asleep and everything is quiet, that cigarette is special.

John: At home nobody smokes. Just in the street or at the door. Anne said that smoking is bad for your sleep.

Paula: This sleep thing is very complicated. Even those who sleep well have their own little habits.

Sleep is like most biological characteristics: one does not fit all!

There is considerable individual variability when it comes to sleep.

There are those who sleep a lot and those who sleep a little, those who never wake up during the night and those who wake up at anything, those who fall asleep quickly and those who take some time to fall asleep.

Besides this, we have our body clocks and there can be differences in that too, both in terms of the "period" of the clock, which can be 24 hours, plus or minus a little, which can be tweaked to function better during the daytime or during the nighttime.

This is a way of saying that there are sleeping champions and sleeping weaklings, night owls and morning larks. All of these are normal, but they all need their own particular balance — that is, each of us should function with what one has.

You cannot ask a Night Owl to wake up early, nor a Lark to be awaken late, nor somebody who needs a lot of sleep to sleep less, or somebody who sleeps lightly to sleep with the window open.

As to the issue of how many hours you should sleep, the answer is simple: 85 to 90% of healthy adults sleep between 7 and 8 hours a night; 5 to 8% need to sleep less than 6h and 5% need to sleep between 9 and 10 hours.

Age also plays its part. According to the National Sleep Foundation[16],[17] the recommended sleep durations are as follows: 14-17 hours for newborns, 12-15 hours for infants, 11-14 hours for toddlers, 10-13 hours for preschoolers, 9-11 hours for school-aged children, and 8-10 hours for teenagers. Seven to 9 hours is recommended for young adults and adults, and 7-8 hours of sleep is recommended for older adults.

In spite of interindividual differences in sleep duration the risks of sleep deprivation are identical across continents and cultures, meaning that sleep need is not dependent from race, climate, latitude or culture.

Adjusting to the rhythm of our body clocks is also important, and this may mean adjusting to conventional schedules, or a little earlier or later.

We are diurnal creatures and as such sleeping during the day is not as effective as sleeping at night, and it can be counterproductive waking up too early, especially before 6am, or going to bed too late.

Our circadian rhythm has a quasi-gaussian distribution with small percentages in the extremes of "morningness" and "eveningness" while most people are average types, that is, their circadian rhythm has a period close to 24h[18].

---

[16]   National Sleep Foundation: Recommended hours by age: https://www.thensf.org/how-many-hours-of-sleep-do-you-really-need/

[17]   Hirshkowitz M, Whiton K, Albert SM, Alessi C, Bruni O, DonCarlos L, Hazen N, Herman J, Adams Hillard PJ, Katz ES, Kheirandish-Gozal L, Neubauer DN, O'Donnell AE, Ohayon M, Peever J, Rawding R, Sachdeva RC, Setters B, Vitiello MV, Ware JC. National Sleep Foundation's updated sleep duration recommendations: final report. Sleep Health. 2015 Dec;1(4):233-243. doi: 10.1016/j.sleh.2015.10.004. Epub 2015 Oct 31. PMID: 29073398.

[18]   Roenneberg T, Kuehnle T, Juda M, Kantermann T, Allebrandt K, Gordijn M, Merrow M. Epidemiology of the human circadian clock. Sleep Med Rev. 2007 Dec;11(6):429-38. doi: 10.1016/j.smrv.2007.07.005. Epub 2007 Nov 1. PMID: 17936039.

Our reaction to coffee is genetically determined and can vary greatly among individuals. It is the same with tobacco. However, both coffee and tobacco have been shown to have negative effects upon sleep.

Alcohol is socially acceptable as a hypnotic agent due to its corresponding ability to induce sleep, but it has negative effects, since sleep becomes lighter, with more chances of snoring and increased sleep apnoeas.

Having an adverse environment or the need to take care of others (children, the elderly, pets, etc.) tends to interrupt sleep and may lead to persistent insomnia.

Whatever our individual differences, everybody needs to take care of their sleep. Sleep has ensured human survival down through the ages. Evolution has perfected the sleep-wakefulness system, transforming it into the optimal, adaptive and multipurpose system which we nowadays possess. As such we cannot ruin it.

Despite the individual differences there are basic scientifically proven rules for sleep and sleep habits.

3. A NAP? YES OR NO

Jamie: I love having a nap. After lunch, that little sleep on the sofa is wonderful. I don't even need to go to my bed. On the sofa, half lying down is so cosy! It's just a pity I can't do it more often.

Paul: If I have a nap I wake up with a headache. It's a no go for me.

Ray: I have a nap every day. They say I am "Dozy", that it is unhealthy, and so on. But that is what animals do! Lions eat and then they have a nice cosy sleep.

Neal: I also don't like it. I get woolly, I wake up without knowing where I am, and I am rather disorientated.

George: I like having a nap. I don't like the fact that nowadays society never stops. It's one big race, never relaxing. A nap gives me strength and energy.

Rod: When I arrive home shattered, starving and ready to have my dinner, while Ellie is getting the food ready, I doze a little.

Jamie: And do you sleep well at night?

Rod: I fall asleep a bit later, but I am so shattered from work that I would sleep no matter what.

Paul: My grandfather is 80 and has a nap every day. Maybe when I am old I will do the same.

The tendency to have a nap is physiological: after lunch there is a relative drop in our temperature and hence a greater tendency to become sleepy.

In healthy individuals, 20 minutes naps are recommended and refreshing; it restores wakefulness and promotes performance and learning[19]. Having a nap is common in many companies in Japan and in the USA, as it is known that this improves the ability to work in the hours afterwards. They are called "Power Naps".

In hot countries, where the midday temperatures are around 104°F or more, having a siesta is an intelligent and suitable thing to do.

A country like Portugal even has an Association for Friends of the Siesta.

Like everything, having a nap has its advantages and disadvantages, and is suitable for some but should be avoided by others.

Who should have a siesta?

Those who enjoy it; workers on night shifts should have a prophylactic nap before a night shift; patients with narcolepsy, since this is followed by a period without any tendency to sleep, and because it is better to sleep in a programmed manner than suddenly falling asleep under inappropriate circumstances; those who think they are going to do without sleep during the following night.

Who should not take a nap?

Those who suffer from insomnia, because they are going to sleep less and worse at night. Patients with epilepsy or sleep-related migraines, since a siesta can set off one of their critical events. Patients who do it to substitute the effects of ineffective treatment for sleep apnoea, since they should be properly treated. Depressed patients, since extensive naps increase depression and nappers are little more likely to develop depression than non-nappers[20].

---

[19] Dhand R, Sohal H. Good sleep, bad sleep! The role of daytime naps in healthy adults. Curr Opin Pulm Med. 2006 Nov;12(6):379-82. doi: 10.1097/01.mcp.0000245703.92311.d0. PMID: 17053484.

[20] Li L, Zhang Q, Zhu L, Zeng G, Huang H, Zhuge J, Kuang X, Yang S, Yang D, Chen Z, Gan Y, Lu Z, Wu C. Daytime naps and depression risk: A meta-analysis of observational studies. Front Psychol. 2022 Dec 15;13:1051128. doi: 10.3389/fpsyg.2022.1051128. PMID: 36591028; PMCID: PMC9798209.

In the elderly, having a nap is questionable. Those who sleep well at night and do not have any cardiovascular problems can have a nap. Elderly people who sleep badly at night should avoid sleeping during the day. There have been some studies that warn of the potential worsening of cardiovascular problems in the elderly during a siesta. Furthermore, daytime napping is associated with increased risks of major cardiovascular events and deaths in those with >6 h of nighttime sleep but not in those sleeping ≤6 h/night[21].

How long should a nap last?

The sleep organization during a nap is similar to night sleep, that is, approximately after 1 hour you are in deep sleep, and after 90 minutes, you go into REM sleep. That is why if you wake up after 1 hour you are confused and disorientated, due to the slowing down of the brain during deep sleep. If you wake up after 90 or 100 minutes you will have had a complete and refreshing sleep cycle. However, this extended siesta will reduce your sleep that night, which will be shorter. Various studies have shown however that a nap of 20 to 30 minutes is more refreshing, and do not have much effect on night sleep[22].

Long naps are however not refreshing, since they are associate with loss of productivity and sleep inertia. Long and frequent naps, particularly in older subjects, are a risk for dementia and

---

[21] Wang C, Bangdiwala SI, Rangarajan S, Lear SA, AlHabib KF, Mohan V, Teo K, Poirier P, Tse LA, Liu Z, Rosengren A, Kumar R, Lopez-Jaramillo P, Yusoff K, Monsef N, Krishnapillai V, Ismail N, Seron P, Dans AL, Kruger L, Yeates K, Leach L, Yusuf R, Orlandini A, Wolyniec M, Bahonar A, Mohan I, Khatib R, Temizhan A, Li W, Yusuf S. Association of estimated sleep duration and naps with mortality and cardiovascular events: a study of 116 632 people from 21 countries. Eur Heart J. 2019 May 21;40(20):1620-1629. doi: 10.1093/eurheartj/ehy695. PMID: 30517670; PMCID: PMC6528160.

[22] Santos-Silva R, Jankavski C, Lorenzi-Filho G. The experience of a Power Nap Center in the largest city of Brazil. Sleep Sci. 2016 Jul-Sep;9(3):151-152. doi: 10.1016/j.slsci.2016.06.006. Epub 2016 Jul 15. PMID: 28123652; PMCID: PMC5241578.

cognitive dysfunction; this relation is bidirectional, since cognitive dysfunction is associated with longer and more frequent naps[23].

What is a good time to take a nap?

A nap should be taken at a normal time, that is around 2pm, when your central temperature goes down a little. Siestas at the end of the day delay night sleep and should be avoided, except when it is necessary to spend the night awake (this is true for both children and adults). Given this, only shift workers or other night workers should have a nap at the end of the day, with the aim of improving their wakefulness during their night work. Patients with narcolepsy should have a siesta before an activity in which it is essential that they stay awake: driving, giving a talk, etc.

Synthesis - A nap is good for some and should be avoided by others. Sleep duration is like a glass of water – you can drink it in one go or sip it, but the total duration always stays the same.

Summertime, the sun burns, and a nap feels good

---

[23] Li P, Gao L, Yu L, Zheng X, Ulsa MC, Yang HW, Gaba A, Yaffe K, Bennett DA, Buchman AS, Hu K, Leng Y. Daytime napping and Alzheimer's dementia: A potential bidirectional relationship. Alzheimers Dement. 2023 Jan;19(1):158-168. doi: 10.1002/alz.12636. Epub 2022 Mar 17. PMID: 35297533; PMCID: PMC9481741.

4. I SLEEP A LITTLE, I SLEEP A LOT

Richard: I've always slept just a little. I'm fine with around 5 or 6 hours of sleep. In the morning I wake up in good spirits, plenty of energy. I don't have difficulty in falling asleep, and I do not wake up at night. I don't have any dreams or nightmares.

Amy: I sleep a lot. My family says I am not normal.

Gloria: Well, she spends her life sleeping. We've all got up and she is in bed. There is no way of getting her out of bed.

Amy: Yes, they think I am a shirker, but it is nothing of the kind. It's just I need to sleep a lot to feel OK. Normally I need at least 10 hours and a little bit more at weekends whenever possible.

Richard: Really?! I go to bed at midnight, 1:00 am and I wake up at 6:00 a.m., ready for a new day. They say you need 8 hours, but I am fine with 5 or 6. Is there something wrong with that? I don't think so.

Amy: Well, if don't get my 10 hours' sleep, I am good for nothing. I mix up words, I am absent minded. Sleepy. But apart from that I am just like you when I sleep, waking up well and my sleep is peaceful. I don't even move. My sheets aren't crumpled, and I almost don't need to make my bed. I don't snore, I don't have nightmares, and I am not depressed. I think that everything is fine with me.

Gloria: I don't know who you take after. You take after your father's family... My family is full of hard-working people. In your father's family there are some poets, who wander around the world going nowhere.

Amy: There you go bugging me! I am not lazy and the "poets" in my father's family are fine people and work hard.

Richard: Don't get angry with each other. Each to his or her own type. Gloria is blonde and Amy is much more brunette, but, besides this, she looks really like you.

Richard is probably a short sleeper.

The short sleepers sleep more efficiently than the others, and keep the so-called "core" sleep stages, that is, slow wave sleep and REM sleep, and spend less time on what is considered as dispensable sleep, that is, stage 2 NREM sleep.

Which are the other short sleepers' characteristics[24]:

> *they usually sleep between 4 to 6 hours,*
> *they do not extend sleep whenever possible (weekends, holidays, etc)*
> *they don't need an alarm clock to wake up*
> *they feel refreshed with their sleep*
> *they are alert and do not complain of sleepiness*
> *they sleep well without difficulties and awakenings*

Short sleep is a physical characteristic, often running in families with some genes involved, namely some intrinsic factors in specific genes like DEC2, NPSR1, mGluR1, and β1-AR mutant genes[25].

Short sleep is not a sign of intelligence or having a peculiar dynamism.

This type of person is to be found at one of the extremes of the normal distribution pattern, which describes the duration of sleep in the normal population and is characteristic of 5 to 8% of the population.

The fact that there are these people who sleep less, but who, when they sleep, sleep well or even really well, does not enable

---

[24] National Sleep Foundation https://www.sleepfoundation.org/how-sleep-works/short-sleeper-syndrome

[25] Yook JH, Rizwan M, Shahid NUA, Naguit N, Jakkoju R, Laeeq S, Reghefaoui T, Zahoor H, Mohammed L. Some Twist of Molecular Circuitry Fast Forwards Overnight Sleep Hours: A Systematic Review of Natural Short Sleepers' Genes. Cureus. 2021 Oct 25;13(10):e19045. doi: 10.7759/cureus.19045. PMID: 34722012; PMCID: PMC8547374.

us to extend the short sleep model to the remaining population. Those who do not have these characteristics will undergo sleep deprivation if they sleep less than needed.

Short sleep and shortening sleep are for social and cultural reasons completely different.

Some famous people have had short sleep. Classic figures are Napoleon, Florence Nightingale, Thomas Edison, and more recently, Madonna and Bill Clinton[26].

Currently there is the idea that genius and successful people have a short sleep. However, many genius and success people sleep normally around 7 to 8 hours a day. Examples: Beethoven, Gates, Bezos, Zuckerberg, Oprah Winfrey, Arianna Huffington, Jimmy Wales, super athletes as Ronaldo, Nadal, Djokovic, Venus Williams

Sleep may be physiologically extended, as in the case of Amy, who represents a long sleeper.

Just as in the case of short sleepers, these individuals are at one of the extremes of the so-called normal distribution pattern and make up around 2% of the population.

Long sleepers feel refreshed upon morning awakening, but they will feel sleepy in case they don't sleep enough. In principle, once other problems have been excluded, such as snoring, hypersomnia, the presence of endocrinological problems, etc., we are dealing here with normal individuals. It is important, however, to have as a gauge that, for an adult, sleeping regularly more than 10 hours a day is in principle abnormal.

---

[26]   https://balancethegrind.co/collections/the-sleeping-habits-routines-of-18-successful-people/
https://thesleepjourney.com/sleeping-habits-of-successful-celebrities/
https://brooklynbedding.com/blog/the-unorthodox-sleep-habits-of-7-famous-people

Individuals who are long sleepers are often considered as being lazy or dreamy, unable to fit into the demands of current working and societal patterns. Such a statement is totally unfair.

The duration of sleep in everyone is an individual characteristic, which is genetically determined.

Famous people who have slept a lot include Darwin, who slept 9h plus a nap, Albert Einstein, the mathematician de Moivre, super athletes Lebron James, Andy Murray and Rodger Federer, but the most famous of all is certainly the Sleeping Beauty.

Shortening sleep should not be a social rule.
Long sleep is not laziness nor stupidity.

5. NOTHING CAN WAKE ME UP

"I set 3 alarm clocks, plus my mobile phone. I ask my mother to call me and nothing. They have even poured water over my head, because removing the covers does nothing. Nothing works. That is my problem."

"Has this always been the case?"

"Well, almost always."

"What is it like during your holidays?"

"Oh, no problems then, everything goes fine."

"What time do you go to bed and get up during the holidays?"

"I go to bed at 2:00 or 3:00 am and get up around midday, 1:00 pm"

"And when you are working, what happens?"

"Well, then I still go to bed at 2:00 or 3:00 am and I get up at 8:00 am because I have to go to work."

"Well, if you only sleep 5 hours, it is natural that you won't be able to wake up. There are three solutions: either wake up later, or go to bed earlier; or do both, getting up a little later and going to bed a little earlier."

"But Doctor, the problem is that I cannot wake up."

"Of course, you cannot with your present lifestyle. You must change it to start waking up normally.

Complaints about not being able to <u>wake up in the morning</u> are often related to bad sleeping habits with short sleep duration.

Sleep duration is genetically limited: you cannot extend it indefinitely, nor reduce it excessively.

Wakefulness duration is also genetically determined for each animal species.

Reducing sleep increases deep sleep, REM sleep and sleep pressure.

Levels of cortisol display a sharp increase immediately upon awakening, known as the cortisol awakening response[27].

Episodes of not being able to wake up may result from a compensatory excess of deep sleep, with its high awakening threshold, increased arousal threshold, from dysfunction in either REM sleep or cognition, poor cortisol awakening response, poor night sleep or poor sensitivity to light.

Despite the somewhat bizarre episodes which can occur, sleep deprivation cases, can be solved with an adjustment of daily sleeping habits.

Distinction must be made in several cases:

- *Idiopathic hypersomnia. In this situation night sleep has persistently a long duration and awakening is difficult with a non-refreshed sleep.*
- *Delayed sleep phase disorder (DSPD)- Difficult awakening at conventional schedules is a key symptom of DSPD; these patients might have an increased arousal threshold and some of them must have REM and /or cognitive abnormalities associated with awakening difficulty[28].*

---

[27] Elder GJ, Ellis JG, Barclay NL, Wetherell MA. Assessing the daily stability of the cortisol awakening response in a controlled environment. BMC Psychol. 2016 Jan 28; 4:3. doi: 10.1186/s40359-016-0107-6. PMID: 26818772; PMCID: PMC4730747.

[28] Solheim B, Olsen A, Kallestad H, Langsrud K, Bjorvatn B, Gradisar M, Sand T. Cognitive performance in DSWPD patients upon awakening from habitual sleep compared with forced conventional sleep. J Sleep Res. 2019 Oct;28(5):e12730. doi: 10.1111/jsr.12730. Epub 2018 Aug 13. PMID: 30105851.

- *Cerebral palsy – difficult morning awakening possibly due to visual impairment and consequent reduction of light stimulation impact[29].*

If you are healthy and sleep the hours you need, you will wake up easily.

[29] Lélis AL, Cardoso MV, Hall WA. Sleep disorders in children with cerebral palsy: An integrative review. Sleep Med Rev. 2016 Dec;30:63-71. doi: 10.1016/j. smrv.2015.11.008. Epub 2015 Dec 11. PMID: 26874066.

6. SLEEP FROM THE NEWBORN BABY TO GRANNY

The Sparrow family is celebrating Granny birthday, she is 80 years old. They joined together Grandpa Roger Sparrow, their son Henry, his wife Mary, the three children Jack, Katie and Daisy and the newborn baby John

At present they are all sleeping well, but remembering old and difficult days they start speaking about their sleep

John, one month old, sleeps quietly most of the time. He wakes up to for breastfeeding, which is quite often and regular, during the day and night, but falls asleep soon after.

He has a polyphasic sleep and is still unable to distinguish between day and night

Granny explained that when is eyes are moving, he is in REM sleep. He is in REM sleep quite often, and soon after falling asleep. Newborns do not have yet slow wave sleep which only occurs around the 3rd month of life.

He is beautiful and healthy and is growing a little bit every day.

Daisy is now five; she makes no longer tantrums to go to bed and does not invade their parents' bed. She is beautiful and smart, learns quite well at the pre-school, and is becoming quite sweet after the ballet lessons.

She has all the sleep stages, slow wave sleep is quite long, and REM sleep is much less prolonged when compared with John. She still likes to nap after lunch, i.e., she has a biphasic sleep.

Katie is a schoolgirl and does not require the after-lunch napping. Her sleep duration is shorter when compared to Daisy's sleep, her slow wave sleep is also slightly shorter.

Jack is an adolescent and is sleep is changing so much as his own body. The limbs are longer so that he looks a little bit clumsy, the beard is appearing and sometimes nobody understands him. He likes to fall asleep later and wake up also later, and this is called the adolescence sleep phase delay. When he exaggerates and falls asleep too late, he falls asleep in the morning class. He is not convinced of long-term benefits; his brain requires immediate rewarding.

Mary is always worried about the children, the housekeeping, and his own work as a teacher. When she is tired, she shouts easily, and she does not sleep well in these special periods of the month, which regularly occur. To prevent her tiredness everybody must help her in the daily routines. She sleeps around 7 hours per night.

Henry is often tired with his work at the Bank, but he usually picks Katie and Jack from school. He does not like children's noise when is listening to the news, but he often cooks the dinner while his wife is taking care of the smallest ones. Mother says he snores after partying with his friends. He likes to cycle with the family during the weekends. He sleeps around 7 to 8 hours per night.

Granny and Grandpa sleep a little less, 6 to 7 hours per night. In both, slow wave sleep and REM are somewhat reduced, and they like to go to bed earlier and wake up earlier too. Grandpa snores a little bit according to Grandma complaints and wakes up once to go to the toilet; they now sleep in separate beds. Grandpa enjoys napping.

Sleep changes markedly across the life span. Duration, sleep stages, circadian characteristics, awakenings and possible sleep

disturbances have specific age-related patterns[30,31,32]. Sleep between

Neonates sleep between 14 and 17h per day, in a polyphasic sleep; they have two types of sleep: Active sleep, which will evolve to REM sleep and Quiet sleep, which will evolve to NREM; the ultradian duration of sleep cycles is 30 to 70 min; sleep spindles and Slow Wave Sleep (SWS) will appear around 3 to 4 months.

Infants sleep between 12 and 15h; the adult sleep stages are well defined but the percentages of REM and SWS are higher.

Toddlers and preschool children will present a progressive decline of TST, WASO, REM sleep and number of sleep cycles, and a progressive increase in sleep cycle duration, sleep stage shifts and N2. For toddlers sleep duration varies between 11 and 14h per day; for preschool children the values are 10 and 13h per day. The polyphasic characteristic reduces also progressively and preschool children have a biphasic sleep.

School children sleep duration varies between 9 and 11h per day

Adolescents sleep duration varies between 8 and 10h per day, and have a phase delay circadian pattern

Adults have a decrease of sleep duration, Sleep efficiency, SWS and REM and increase N1 and WASO; sleep duration varies between 7 and 9h per day

[30] Mutti C, Misirocchi F, Zilioli A, Rausa F, Pizzarotti S, Spallazzi M, Parrino L. Sleep and brain evolution across the human lifespan: A mutual embrace. Front Netw Physiol. 2022 Aug 3;2:938012. doi: 10.3389/fnetp.2022.938012. PMID: 36926070; PMCID: PMC10013002.

[31] Logan RW, McClung CA. Rhythms of life: circadian disruption and brain disorders across the lifespan. Nat Rev Neurosci. 2019 Jan;20(1):49-65. doi: 10.1038/s41583-018-0088-y. PMID: 30459365; PMCID: PMC6338075.

[32] 4Miner B, Kryger MH. Sleep in the Aging Population. Sleep Med Clin. 2017 Mar;12(1):31-38. doi: 10.1016/j.jsmc.2016.10.008. Epub 2016 Dec 20. PMID: 28159095; PMCID: PMC5300306.

**Elderly** have a further decrease of sleep duration (6 to 8h), Sleep efficiency, SWS and REM and increase in N1, WASO and sleep disorders prevalence (insomnia, sleep apnoea, periodic limb movements of sleep, REM Behaviour disorder and sleep disturbances associated with medical and neurologic disorders). Sleep microstructure changes since K complexes and sleep spindles decrease in amplitude and density. Circadian alterations do occur with a tendency to have an advanced sleep phase pattern and a biphasic sleep and a lower amplitude melatonin rhythm.

Sleep varies markedly across the lifespan

C. What is a bad Sleep?

1. SLEEPING TOO LITTLE

MY PROBLEM? I DON'T SLEEP

Life is going well, but I cannot sleep. It's been like this for several years. Perhaps it started after my son's accident. A difficult period... Until then I slept well, but then my insomnia little by little started to get worse.

I've stopped drinking coffee and I have a light dinner, but it always happens the same. I go to bed early because, if I do not, it is even worse, and I have more time to sleep.

I am allergic to my bed. As soon as I lie down it triggers my insomnia and I stay wide awake for hours.

I really try and force myself to sleep because I know that it is bad just to sleep a little, but I look at the clock and I have only slept for 1 hour. It is 4 am and I cannot fall back asleep. The time passes by, and I cannot sleep, and with every passing hour I will have less time to sleep.

Sleepless nights are worrying. I think it's my karma because I was like that as a child. Sleeping in a bed is beyond me, but on the sofa with the television on, I can easily fall asleep. As soon as I go to bed, puff !!!, sleep goes away ...

I don't have any problems in life, and I don't feel depressed. I do not like taking pills, but I know that I cannot live sleeping so little.

This is a chronic primary insomnia, previously called psychophysiological insomnia. The complaint is chronic (duration longer than 3 months and frequency higher than 3 times per week); patient has sleep initiation or maintenance problems, adequate opportunity and circumstances to sleep and daytime consequences[33,34].

The main problem of patients is centred on sleep, on their incapacity and worry that they are unable to sleep and the fear of the associated consequences.

Insomnia generally starts from a problem which has occurred in one's life, but then tends to drag on independently of such problem. It is more common in women.

Patients have a horrible fear/worry of not sleeping and face the moment they lie down with anxiety. They make desperate efforts to sleep, but the more they try and the greater their fear, the less they sleep. Often at night they take their problems to bed and "chew over" their daily affairs.

The sleeping medications for these patients have paradoxical effects and may not be effective. Many have the habit of gradually increasing the dose to keep up the effect.

Treatment is, however, possible, and involves behavioural and pharmacological therapies, once the problem has been understood by the patient. In these cases, cognitive behavioural therapies are currently recognised as being more effective in the long term[35].

Although each case is "a case", there are general rules to bear in mind:

[33] Sateia MJ. International classification of sleep disorders-third edition: highlights and modifications. Chest. 2014 Nov;146(5):1387-1394. doi: 10.1378/chest.14-0970. PMID: 25367475.

[34] Kaur H, Spurling BC, Bollu PC. Chronic Insomnia. 2023 Jul 10. In: StatPearls [Internet]. Treasure Island (FL): StatPearls Publishing; 2024 Jan–. PMID: 30252392.

[35] Buysse DJ. Insomnia. JAMA. 2013 Feb 20;309(7):706-16. doi: 10.1001/jama.2013.193. PMID: 23423416; PMCID: PMC3632369.

In the morning:

- Do morning exercise, such as walking for around 30 minutes.
- Sit out in the sun in the morning.

During the day:

- Take regular breaks at work.
- Choose relaxation techniques and/or regular massages.
- Don't work until you go to bed.
- Avoid coffee and other stimulants.
- Try just to do what you are capable of. Forget perfection and be "reasonable and kind" to yourself.
- Don't eat too late and avoid heavy foods.

After dinner:

- Don't fall asleep watching television.
- Don't watch TV in bed.
- Have a time when you organise your things for the next day, and write them down on a piece of paper or in a diary.
- Take a moment just for yourself.
- Avoid very brightly lit places.
- Do not do any important physical activities.
- There are certain activities that can help: a small walk, a glass of warm or hot milk; a warm bath.

Going to bed and sleeping:

- Don't go to bed too early, and don't spend hours in bed waiting to fall asleep.
- Don't sleep with the window or the blinds or curtains open.
- Don't have any light in the room.
- Choose a pleasant temperature which is not too hot or too cold.

- *Avoid noise – if there is noise outside, double glazing may help. If your husband (or wife) snores, earplugs may help.*
- *Take any clocks out of the room or turn the luminous dials to the wall.*
- *If you are awake do not clock watch.*
- *Do not make any effort to fall asleep. If you cannot sleep, it is better to get up and do something pleasant in a low-lit ambience and only go back to bed when you feel sleepy again.*
- *Do not worry about waking up in the middle of the night. There are periods of the night when it is impossible to fall asleep. It is as if the "sleep gates" have been closed. What this means is that you cannot fall asleep at a specific hour, but if you let this pass without worrying then a little later, you can fall asleep easily.*

In your daily routine:

- *When you have more tasks than you can do, either ask for help or simplify them.*
- *Be optimistic.*

If you suffer from insomnia do not give in to it. It can be treated.

2. SLEEPING BADLY

I STOP BREATHING, I THINK I AM GOING TO DIE

I wake up distressed in the middle of the night, without being able to breathe. My heart is racing and I'm all sweaty with the sensation that I am going to leave this world.

It's a terrible sensation.

My wife is really distressed without knowing what to do. She gives me a glass of water and it passes. It's scary.

Then we lie down again, and I calmly go back to sleep.

She also says I snore.

I heard a story about a friend of mine that I think is different: something similar happens and then he gets so nervous he can't fall asleep. But my friend has similar episodes during the day, when he finds himself in enclosed spaces or places with a lot of people.

I don't think I'm as nervous as him.

This episode is probably a nocturnal suffocation crisis, more recently called Paroxysmal Nocturnal Dyspnoea[36].

It can present just as in this case: Suffocation, tachycardia and the sensation of death, which go away with a glass of water, and the patient goes back to sleep. It does not require treatment, but it is important to relax such patients and verify through tests that they do not have apnoeas during sleep, since snoring also exists.

This may also occur during sleep apnoeas, and in that case, the individuals snore and have other symptoms of apnoeas. Patients have such a lack of air that they may have run to the window

---

[36]   Paroxysmal Nocturnal Dyspnea Causes and Treatment (healthline.com)

to breathe better (nocturnal asphyxia)[37]. *If this is the case, this requires urgent treatment.*

It may eventually be a symptom of heart failure, which more often is felt as a difficulty of breath when lying down (orthopnea).

It may also be a panic attack[38]. *In this case, patients will not go back to sleep, but remain anxious, afraid of dying and having similar episodes during the day and/or other signs of panic. This implies psychologic or psychiatric treatment.*

It may be a laryngospasm, a situation which is accompanied by a dry noise due to the spasm of the larynx. Patients must be observed by an ENT specialist.

If you wake up suffocating, you have to know what is behind it.

[37] Ayas NT, Hirsch AA, Laher I, Bradley TD, Malhotra A, Polotsky VY, Tasali E. New frontiers in obstructive sleep apnoea. Clin Sci (Lond). 2014 Aug;127(4):209-16. doi: 10.1042/CS20140070. PMID: 24780001; PMCID: PMC4348094.

[38] Levitan MN, Nardi AE. Nocturnal panic attacks: clinical features and respiratory connections. Expert Rev Neurother. 2009 Feb;9(2):245-54. doi: 10.1586/14737175.9.2.245. PMID: 19210198.

3. SLEEPING TOO MUCH

THEY SAY I AM A SLEEPYHEAD

How is today going to be? I need to think...

Yesterday I fell asleep at the hairdresser. At least they all know about me. I started dreaming immediately. About what? Well, I just don't recall, something that had happened.

I fell asleep while she was cutting my hair!

"Mrs Brown, wake up! I might cut off your ear."

A lady who did not know me burst out laughing. So be it. I must hurry up to get off to work.

Peter is taking me. He's afraid I'll just fall asleep unwittingly on the metro.

Peter, are you ready?

Let's go...

Margaret, wake up, we're there. Be careful. Don't fall and hurt yourself. I'll pick you up at 5:00 pm See you later...

(Horn sounds)

What a fright! Margaret, you were about to be run over. Are you alright? You've dropped your bag. Get up.

What happened?

"Mrs, you fell!"

"It's nothing, everything's fine."

"Are you really, OK?"

"Yes, it's gone. I don't think I lost anything. The honking scared me."

"Of course I honked. You looked like a sleepwalker crossing the street. Are you alright? Did you faint?"

No I didn't faint. I lost my energy. I've been tired but I'm alright now.

Goodbye, Peter. See you later. Everything's OK.

Look, here comes Mrs Jones. I'm going to meet her.

"So Mrs Brown did it happen again?"

"Yes, imagine, I was crossing the road and some stupid idiot honked. I got scared and fell."

"It's very dangerous. You simply must go to the doctor!"

"I've been. First they said it was epilepsy, now it's depression. They gave me some pills and it seems they don't know what's the matter with me. They say I'm a sleepyhead, but these falls are the worst. That's when I get scared. The other day it was like being in a joke.

I felt my eyes closing, my head falling and my knees buckling. They say I'm a sleepyhead, Mrs Jones, that I can't control myself as it is stronger than me, but if I sleep a little, I feel better."

"Let it go, Mrs Brown, it is better like that. You sleep a lot and night time must be wonderful. Not like me. It's nearly impossible for me to fall asleep."

"Come again? Well at night, Mrs Jones, I don't sleep well. I dream and toss and turn. The other day I woke up and couldn't move. I see strange things when I fall asleep, but I know I am not mad. I don't even tell my husband as I'm afraid he'll think it ridiculous.

They said it was epilepsy but after all I'm not epileptic. I don't understand any of this.

This has been going on for 37 years and I don't see a way out of it. So many doctors, so many remedies and nothing worked."

Mrs Brown suffers from Narcolepsy with cataplexy, a disorder characterized by:

- *Sleepiness during the day, with irresistible microsleep episodes, and frequent dreams. The microsleep episodes are remedial and stop you from falling back asleep in the hours immediately afterwards.*
- *Cataplexy, that is, periods with a lack of force, without loss of the senses, set off by an emotion or scare (honking, joke, etc.).*

In these episodes parts of the body gradually droop: eyelids, neck, knees, hands and this may result in a complete fall.

- *Sleep paralysis, i.e., waking up at night and not being able to move.*
- *Hypnagogic hallucinations, seeing or feeling strange things, sometimes threatening or scary, when falling asleep.*
- *There is a tendency for weight to increase.*

Narcolepsy is a disorder which effects 2 to 4.7 out of 10 000 people, and as such has a similar rate of prevalence to Multiple Sclerosis. The prevalence varies across countries, and it is higher in Japan and lower in Israel.

Many are certainly badly diagnosed, either because they do not go to a doctor or because when they do, it is not diagnosed.

It is known that in these patients an immunological insult affects the orexin (or hypocretin) system, with a pronounced reduction of this neurotransmitter in the Central Nervous System, due to destruction of the orexin producing cells in the hypothalamus.

It is a disorder which is sometimes hereditary, linked to the HLA system, with most patients having the HLA DQB60102 or HLA DQA10102 genotype.

Diagnosis is carried out through a clinical history, which may contain only some of the symptoms described, as well as ancillary diagnostic tests. The linking of sleepiness and cataplexy is enough to make the diagnosis of Narcolepsy with cataplexy or Narcolepsy type 1, according to the recent International Classification of Sleep Disorders[39].

The essential tests are a nocturnal polysomnography followed by a multiple sleep latency test the next day; lumbar puncture for quantification of orexin levels in the liquor is a further step: in narcolepsy orexin levels are very low.

At night the patient has insomnia and a reduction in the latency of REM sleep. The multiple sleep latency test proves the sleepiness (the mean sleep latency is lower than 8 minutes) and the REM sleep anomalies, with at least 2 sleep onset REM episodes during the test.

Narcolepsy often starts in adolescence with one or several symptoms but does not get much worse during the patient's life.

The most incapacitating aspects are excessive sleepiness and cataplexy, which hampers one's social life and may lead to accidents. The fact that it starts at young ages implies that it is a lifelong chronic condition, with harmful effects on the quality of life.

There are no important intellectual or cognitive effects.

---

[39] Sateia MJ. International classification of sleep disorders-third edition: highlights and modifications. Chest. 2014 Nov;146(5):1387-1394. doi: 10.1378/chest.14-0970. PMID: 25367475.

Even though there are hereditary factors, the risk of transmission to children is small, due to the low prevalence of the genes. As a general rule it "jumps" a generation.

There are treatment rules.

- *Acceptance of the disorder and of the required changes in life.*
- *Good lifestyle hygiene, with prophylactic naps. It is better to sleep in a programmed manner than to fall asleep without wishing to.*
- *Treating sleepiness with medication. Nowadays there are effective treatments, specifically modafinil, pitolisant, armodafinil, and sodium oxybate, which is also used to treat insomnia and cataplexy)[40]. New drugs, such as, oral orexin receptor 2-selective agonists and others, are nowadays appearing on the market.*
- *Cataplexy is treated with appropriate drugs, specifically certain antidepressants and, more recently, with sodium oxybate and its extended release formulation.*
- *Treat the insomnia.*

If you suffer from narcolepsy, don't just pass it off as being a "sleepyhead" or lazy".

It can be treated, and you can improve the quality of your life.

---

[40] Maski K, Trotti LM, Kotagal S, Robert Auger R, Rowley JA, Hashmi SD, Watson NF. Treatment of central disorders of hypersomnolence: an American Academy of Sleep Medicine clinical practice guideline. J Clin Sleep Med. 2021 Sep 1;17(9):1881-1893. doi: 10.5664/jcsm.9328. PMID: 34743789; PMCID: PMC8636351.

4. MOVING A LOT

I DON'T FIND MY SLEEP POSITION

- My sleep it quite unrestful. To fall asleep and take a lot of time ... 1 or 2 hours at least.
- Since sleep does not come easily, I get irritated and turn to the right, turn to the left, put myself on the back, try the belly afterwards and sleep does not come.

  I go out of bed and do something useful but when I return the same restlessness occurs, and I look desperately for an adequate position. I don't find my sleep position.
- Do you have strange feelings or unpleasant sensations in your arms or legs?
- No, not at all it is mostly the anxiety and the need to find a position. Afterwards I have no time left to sleep properly and my sleep is curtailed. Furthermore, if it happens, I awake during the night the same drama occurs: an endless tragedy to find a proper sleep position. I start listening to everything, my heart beats fast and I can feel my heart beating at the pillow; it beats fast! The noise of my husband breathing is very disturbing, and I will hear a fly in case it will came to our room.

  The morning, I am not tired, I am really exhausted of all this turning around during the night.

We all require a comfortable sleep position and each one as its preferred position during sleep onset. Some prefer to lay to the right, other to the left, others choose to lay down on their back while others only achieve sleep whenever laying on their belly.

Many mammals have the same problems and dogs turn around before laying down while cats opt for the most comfortable position in the most comfortable place.

However, during the night, we change position several times; this number varies across ages, children move more than adults, and among individuals, some have a quieter sleep than others.

However, for some persons sleep onset position may become a drama. Some are anxious and the sleep related anxiety prevents them of being still; some others may move because they have pain, mostly musculoskeletal pain, which increases in a fixed position; however, in some others the restlessness is associated with restless legs syndrome or restless sleep disorder[41].

The mechanisms behind restlessness may be due to low ferritin, excessive sympathetic activity, neuropsychiatric dysfunction or events occurring during sleep associated with arousals, such as sleep apnoea, bruxism, hypoxemias etc.

In children restless sleep may have multiple causes, namely, sleep-disordered breathing, adenotonsillectomy, respiratory disorders, otitis media, smoke exposure, sleep-related movement disorders[42] (restless legs, periodic limb movements and bruxism), restless sleep disorder, NREM parasomnias[43], neurologic or psychiatric disorders

---

[41] DelRosso LM, Silvestri R, Ferri R. Restless Sleep Disorder. Sleep Med Clin. 2021 Jun;16(2):381-387. doi: 10.1016/j.jsmc.2021.03.003. PMID: 33985662.

[42] DelRosso LM, Mogavero MP, Ferri R. Restless sleep disorder, restless legs syndrome, and periodic limb movement disorder-Sleep in motion! Pediatr Pulmonol. 2022 Aug;57(8):1879-1886. doi: 10.1002/ppul.25305. Epub 2021 Mar 1. PMID: 33527761.

[43] Senel GB, Kochan Kizilkilic E, Karadeniz D. Restless sleep disorder in children with NREM parasomnias. Sleep. 2021 Jul 9;44(7):zsab049. doi: 10.1093/sleep/zsab049. PMID: 33630032.

such as sleep related epilepsy[44] *and **ADHD**[45], neurodevelopmental disorders such as **Down syndrome**, other sleep disorders*[46].

If restlessness impinges upon your sleep or upon your sleep onset check for the causes!

---

[44] Benbir Senel G, Tunali A, Karadeniz D, DelRosso LM. Restless sleep disorder in children with epileptic and non-epileptic nocturnal attacks. J Sleep Res. 2024 Feb;33(1):e13963. doi: 10.1111/jsr.13963. Epub 2023 Jun 15. PMID: 37318087.

[45] Kapoor V, Ferri R, Stein MA, Ruth C, Reed J, DelRosso LM. Restless sleep disorder in children with attention-deficit/hyperactivity disorder. J Clin Sleep Med. 2021 Apr 1;17(4):639-643. doi: 10.5664/jcsm.8984. PMID: 33155540; PMCID: PMC8020699.

[46] DelRosso LM, Picchietti DL, Spruyt K, Bruni O, Garcia-Borreguero D, Kotagal S, Owens JA, Simakajornboon N, Ferri R; International Restless Legs Syndrome Study Group (IRLSSG). Restless sleep in children: A systematic review. Sleep Med Rev. 2021 Apr;56:101406. doi: 10.1016/j.smrv.2020.101406. Epub 2020 Dec 1. PMID: 33341437.

5. Making odd sounds

MY GIRLFRIEND CANNOT STAND MY SNORING

— You know ... my life changed recently. I divorced two years ago and recently I have a new relation which seems quite promising, since we go along quite well. She is younger, somewhat younger, but we are quite close.

However, I have a problem: she complains about my snoring My ex-wife also complained but we never solved the problem I heard snoring might impact upon sexual performance and upon couples' relations and I am worried.

— Did your father snore or someone in your family?

— Yes, indeed my father snored like a horse and my son also snores. My own snoring is longstanding ...

— Do you drink alcoholic beverages at dinner or after it

— No by no means, I strongly reduced alcohol; nowadays it is restricted to social occasions

— And about weight and physical activity?

— I practise sports regularly, tennis and golf. I am in a good shape and my weight is controlled

— Do you have other health problems: high blood pressure, arrhythmia, etc?

— No, I made a check-up recently and everything was OK.

— I will ask you about sleep apnoea related symptoms ...

Snoring is a respiratory noise, which occurs during sleep, and is associated with tone oscillations. It can occur in all ages, since birth and is always a sign of a difficult breathing, i.e., a difficult flow in the upper airway. Snoring prevalence increases with age and is higher in males (35–45%) than females (15–28%).

It may be or not associated with sleep apnoea, but even when occurring independently it heralds the possibility of apnoea occurrence somewhere in the future. Other risks imply matrimonial

disputes and cardiovascular, cognitive, sexual dysfunctions, daytime sleepiness, reduced energy/vitality, daytime anxiety, risk of depression, stress, and fatigue.

Snoring implies a restriction or even obstruction in the upper airway, which increases its resistance to the air circulation during breathing; the vibration of the soft tissues is responsible for the audible noise.

The provoked vibration in the soft tissues induces a localized neuropathy due to its chronic evolution[47].

The causes vary.

- *It can occur in cases of nasal obstruction, due to any problem at the nose (inflammatory disorders, septal deviation, etc)*
- *It can occur in cases of mouth breathing, in patients with either a reduced lumen of the upper airway or an obstruction in the transition from the Oro to the nasopharynx*
- *It can supervene in cases of specific facial configuration, such as, a bird-like face with a small maxilla an a prominent nose or in cases of oval face associated with a small maxilla or in cases of a long face and a long neck*
- *it can also exist in abnormal facial conformation due to congenital disorders (Pierre Robin, etc)*
- *It is also quite frequent in persons who are obese or overweight and in those with a large neck*
- *A genetic predisposition I clear, with heritability estimates suggesting that 18–28% of variance can be accounted for by genetic factors and some genes have been identified (Gene-based associations identify 173 genes, including*

47 Patel JA, Ray BJ, Fernandez-Salvador C, Gouveia C, Zaghi S, Camacho M. Neuromuscular function of the soft palate and uvula in snoring and obstructive sleep apnea: A systematic review. Am J Otolaryngol. 2018 May-Jun;39(3):327-337. doi: 10.1016/j.amjoto.2018.03.006. Epub 2018 Mar 5. PMID: 29525140.

DLEU7, MSRB3 and POC5, highlighting genes expressed in the brain, cerebellum, lungs, blood and oesophagus)[48].
- *Lifestyles are also important, namely heavy and late meals, alcoholic beverages at dinner or before bedtime, idem for sedatives and benzodiazepines and smoking*
- *Sleep posture is quite important, namely supine position (sleep on the back)*

The solution depends on complaints and patient characteristics.

Snoring can be solved by losing weight, abolishing alcoholic beverages in the evening as well as sleep medication impacting upon breathing and avoiding supine sleep position.

In other cases, nasal surgery might be useful.

Mandibular advancement is often an option and other ENT interventions must be considered whenever reduction of the transition from the nasal to the oropharynx is present.

The male attitudes concerning complaints about their snoring vary a lot. Some do not believe, since they sleep soundly and don't ear whatsoever; others consider snoring is likely since they ear themselves snoring upon falling asleep; others are really concerned about any inconvenience to the bed partner related to snoring and wish efficient solutions.

The attitudes of females are quite different: usually they don't like to snore since "it is a male thing"; so often, they don't believe their husbands, but they might believe their grandsons whenever snoring stars at menopause.

---

[48] Campos AI, García-Marín LM, Byrne EM, Martin NG, Cuéllar-Partida G, Rentería ME. Insights into the aetiology of snoring from observational and genetic investigations in the UK Biobank. Nat Commun. 2020 Feb 14;11(1):817. doi: 10.1038/s41467-020-14625-1. PMID: 32060260; PMCID: PMC7021827.

The bedpartners attitudes also vary. Big concerns around bedpartners health, awake all night to oblige him/her to change body position, ear plugs, discomfort and insomnia, unacceptable requiring independent bed or separate rooms, divorce due to the resulting conflicts

Snoring must be treated and solved!

Laugh and the world laughs with you, snore and you sleep alone.
Anthony Burgess

Strange behaviours

YOU WERE WALKING AROUND THE HOUSE

"You were doing it again today!"

"What?..."

"You went to the living room and to the bathroom and I woke up in time to stop you going to the stairs."

"Yes... I have a vague idea I was doing something... What did I do?"

"You were in the living room and you had already opened the bathroom door. Your eyes were glazed over and you were walking around the table. I don't know how you didn't break the vase! But no... you went around again and didn't touch it.

The worst thing is you went towards the stairs. It was your father, who was working until late, who caught you and brought you back to bed."

"And what did I say?"

"You grunted something, which wasn't understandable, hum... hum... hum...

I said to you "Go to bed", but you went towards the stairs. And that's what scares me, that you could fall and hurt yourself like the last time. I have been so worried, but your father said that he was also like that and it went away. But I think you must go to the doctor."

"Is there any bread? I've got to hurry up and get off to school."

"The bread is right in front of you! You're still asleep. Here's your milk and cereals. Don't spill the glass, see if you are awake. What do you have today?"

"Hum... French... Mathematics...no, it's Art and Design. Today is Wednesday, isn't it?"

"Of course it's Wednesday, now see if you are awake.

You've already spilt the milk. What a drag.

Are you alright?"

"Yes, of course I am."

"You've got to go to the doctor before you hurt yourself. What do I care if you father also used to be like this."

"I'm taking you to the doctor, this is sleepwalking."

"What sleepwalking! It's called somnambulism."

"If it's somnambulism, somnambulists walk while sleeping..."

"Now hurry up so you don't get there late. I'm going to arrange an appointment. The other times you "sleepwalked" you had fever, but not last night, and I think we should find out what is going on."

"It's nothing mum, don't you see that I did 4 hours of sport yesterday. We had a special training session. It must have been that!"

Somnambulism or sleepwalking[49], is in fact a familiar disease which mainly affects boys. It has its own age period, between 8 and 12, and tends to disappear in adult life, but may arise as soon as a child has started to walk.

Nocturnal episodes of sleepwalking occur around 1 hour after falling asleep, when leaving deep sleep.

Sleepwalkers go around the house in a relatively coordinated manner but can also bump into objects and hurt themselves

---

49   Arnulf I. Sleepwalking. Curr Biol. 2018 Nov 19;28(22):R1288-R1289. doi: 10.1016/j. cub.2018.09.062. Epub 2018 Nov 19. PMID: 30458142.

mainly by falling down the stairs, opening a window and stepping out through it. Other behaviours may occur, namely, sit up in bed, scream, speak, swear or mumble, stand up, run, text, search in drawers or handle objects.

The "sleepy state" is in line with the lack of full awareness and responsiveness, mental confusion, inappropriate emotion and/or dreamlike mentation. The sleepwalker maintains a certain memory of what has happened and is capable of having the notion that "something happened"

The risks of an accident are real and must be completely avoided.

Sleepwalking episodes may be activated by fever and by physical exercise but may also occur without any apparent reason.

It is a myth to consider that it is dangerous to wake up a sleepwalker. On the contrary, the sleepwalker should be gently brought back to bed, although in some cases this might result in a violent reaction.

One way of avoiding these episodes is to sleep in a sleeping bag, since the effort of opening the zipper makes the sleepwalker awaken.

It is always important to avoid accidents with windows, doors, ladders, mirrors, glass, etc.

Treatment is only justified in cases with many frequent episodes and may involve the use of paroxetine, benzodiazepine or psychotherapy.

It is important to clarify that, whenever there are different factors to those mentioned above, that is, when there is no family history, when the episodes occur at any hour of the night, or can be repeat twice or several times in the same night, and when, after the episodes, there is a total amnesia or headaches, fatigue and *generalized muscle pain, the aetiology needs to be investigated. There may be other parasomnias or nocturnal epilepsy.*

The nocturnal sleepwalking episodes can be a result of pathologies different from sleepwalker.

Sleepwalking requires protective measures. Not all sleepwalking is due to somnambulism

6. UNCOMMON HOURS TO SLEEP

WEEKENDS PARTIES END AT 6AM

— I am very concerned with him. He was a brilliant student during high school and nowadays he fails, year after year, without seeming to take much care out of it.

— That is your opinion, mine is different

— His friends are all the same, one or two manage to do something, but most are like him, failing classes, giving up the university, engaging in a life without objectives

— The objectives of a carrier or a stable employment are not necessarily the only ones possible. In any case employment is not currently available and lifestyles changed tremendously. Things are not the same anymore.

— You are failing classes or not?

— Yes, more or less

— Well better stop this arguing; could you then explain me your schedules during the week and the weekends.

— What do you mean?

— I mean the hours you wake up, take your breakfast, go to the university, lunch, finish classes, exercise, study, party with friends, play with the computer, have dinner, what do you do after dinner and at what time you go to bed and fell asleep.

There was a silence as if some complex issue was at stake. The boy, in his twenties, looked at me in a vague indecision. His hair was out of order, the clothes also.

— Well! my wake-up hours vary, so it is difficult to say

— Could you give me the range? Between what and what?

— He awakes up always late; the weekends are terrible.

— Shall I ask your mother to leave us alone for some time? Would you mind leaving us alone?

The boy was pleased, and I could start collecting the schedules during the week and the weekends, the meals, the presence at classes, the computer time for studying and fun, the high frequency of sms, the lack of any relevant physical activity, the group of friends, the cannabis and alcohol intake, smoking habits and the disco parties until 6 or 7 am.

So, it means that every weekend, Friday and Saturday, besides the cannabis, the shots and other alcoholic beverages you go to bed 5 hours later relative to weekdays and Sunday you have a big difficulty falling asleep, and your day goes on between your bed and the coach for some TV viewing.

Monday is a difficult day and Tuesday you wake up early and go to bed around 1 or 2 am until Friday and the weekend programming

— More or less, yes...

This boy has a chronic social jet lag, to which it adds the cannabis and the alcohol and the late schedules, even during weekdays.

The risks and dangers of these weekend parties are, indeed, many[50]:

- *Drinking too much alcohol (binge drinking)*
- *Driving after drinking*
- *Unprotected or non-consensual sex*
- *Drink spiking*
- *Drug overdose or alcohol poisoning*
- *Getting into a fight*
- *Getting injured*
- *Social media problems (such as photos of drunken or sexual behavior)*
- *Unsupervision and gate crashing*
- *Being arrested*

[50] Partying safely - Better Health Channel

Furthermore, these behaviours have a greater risk of depression, academic failure and unsuccessful career. The familiar conflicts are frequent due to the difficulty of handling and understanding these problems. The difficulty in decision making is clear, suggesting some impact in executive functions.

The remaining issues are like other circadian dysfunctions.

The treatment is difficult with high failure rates. It implies circadian readjustment, together with behavioural therapy and dependence treatment.

If you live East Coast and go to bed during weekends at 6/7 am it is equivalent to a weekend "travelling" from New York to San Francisco and return.

This practise in reality would be extremely tiring, so don't be surprised for your tiredness!

D. Importance of daily habits: Good and Bad Routines

Nowadays the societal organization, both in terms of work and pleasure, does not comply with the Sleep Needs.
Work schedules, in many countries, tend to start early and end late
Shift work is more common everywhere
Traffic at rush hours implies time stolen to the needed rest
Work stress is worldwide disseminated and frequent
Family meals tend to be substituted by fast food and snacks, at latter times or without regular schedules
Coffee, alcohol are available everywhere
Tobacco and drugs are easily reachable
Electronic gadgets entered many homes and are available since early ages
TV programs go on around the 24hours
Mobile phones and messages give no rest at night
Youngster's amusements go on until morning hours
Sleep medications are presented as formal solutions

And most of all
The present cultures envisage sleep as a waste of time

But
It is known that adequate daily habits are essential both for health and sleep

Indeed
It is known that some habits are terrible for your sleep:
    Irregular meals schedules, late dinner and poor nutrition
    Too much time at home or in bed
    Too much time sitting
    Having nothing to do, no interests and no responsibilities
    Feeling lonely

However
The same Habits might be good or bad depending both on the individuals and the circumstances

1. I KEEP A MEDITERRANEAN DIET

The annual arrangement of the North Star companions' lunch was settled for Sunday. The restaurant was at the seacoast, in a very beautiful beach with wild waves and fantastic dunes

Henry, Marcus, Miriam, Sally, Victor and Amelia were going. Each one followed different direction in their lives and they were curious to know about each other.

Henry was an informatic engineer with a successful career in a Telecommunication company. Married, two sons; his wife could not come.

Marcus transformed the small civil construction firm inherited from his father in a multinational firm, he was building roads and bridges in USA, Canada and South America. Three marriages, two sons, he should bring the new wive, Louise.

Miriam was an executive in a lawyer's firm, dealing mostly with heritages and divorces. Divorced, one daughter.

Sally was a schoolteacher, married with Roger. They have 3 children 2 girls and 1 boy.

Victor was a civil servant of Internal Affairs. Still married despite many girlfriends.

Amelia oversaw with her husband, Simon, her family properties dealing with agriculture products. They had four sons, 2 boys, 2 girls.

At present they are quite different, but in old days they made fantastic camping's in most different and remote places oriented by the "North Star".

The menu decision has been made previously by Amelia, who tried to fit the tastes and choices of each member. It was a difficult job!

Miriam in her daily life used mostly processed food, since did not like cooking. Marcus was a gourmet, used to international food but Louise, his wife was vegan. Henry ate often burgers and got some extra pounds. Sally and Roger had no special preferences, and herself and Simon enjoyed meet or fish in well-cooked recipes.

Lunch began pleasantly. Louise, the newcomer, was young and pretty, with amusing jokes. It was her who started the food discussion

— I cannot understand why, with all the present knowledge, you go on eating meat and fish.

Simon looks at her seriously

— Do you know that hunting started before agriculture?
— Yes, I know, but nowadays we are no longer in prehistoric times, and we presently know the enormous pollution of big cattle herds.

Henry tried to decrease the approach of a fierce discussion

— Well, my Dear, we are like lions and tigers, predators and carnivores. It is a rule of Nature.

Miriam came in his help.

— Dear Louise, I am always eating either processed food or food entering by my car window, so this fantastic menu chosen by Amelia, well cooked, with multiple ingredients and regional dishes seems fantastic.
— Thanks Miriam, I am happy you are enjoying my choice. I did not forget you, Louise, and ordered salads and a vegetarian dish

Louise felt she should stop.

— Amelia thanks everything is perfect. I apologize.

But Sally came back to the point

— I think that with the climate crisis and the technologic development we should take into consideration the herds pollution and the way animals, both cattle and poultry, are treated for producing meat, milk, eggs, etc.
— Both pollution and animal care deserve discussion. Basically, we must discuss whether the present practices are needed for food production around the world — went on Roger

Simon used his experience in agriculture.

— I don't see how we can produce large amounts of food without fertilizers and big cattle herds
— A new agriculture is emerging. In some years everything is going to change — added Roger

Marcus — Nowadays she is always against my gourmet habits, so once in awhile I also eat vegan

Sally looked at Marcus, marvelled with his wife discussion, and felt the danger of an ugly dispute. She changed the subject.

— I think the important issue is to know what a good diet is. There are so many diets nowadays[51] that people no longer know what to do or what to eat.

---

[51] Your Dietary Roadmap: A Comprehensive Guide to 11 Types of Diets (healthynbetter.com)

Miriam — Indeed there are: the Ketogenic diet[52], the Paleo diet[53], Atkins diet, Vegan diet, Intermittent Fasting[54], Zone Diet, Weight Watchers diet, Low carb, Gluten Free, DASH diet

Sally — You are forgetting the Mediterranean Diet

Miriam — Oh yes, indeed, you are right

Roger — You know, since we are both schoolteachers, we must study this nutrition business very well in order to teach and discuss it with our students; we must stop the obesity epidemic which is so deleterious for health and for sleep.

Amelia - Do you feel healthy Louise? Do you sleep well?

Victor - using his playboy abilities — She is so pretty she certainly sleeps well

Louise - I feel healthy, yes. I take great care with nutrients that may miss in a vegan diet, such as, vitamin B12, iron, calcium, omega-3 fatty acids, and zinc. But I never slept well.

Sally — You never sleep well?

Louise — I have been bullied since my childhood either because I was vegan or because I was an animal defender activist. So vegan yes, good sleeper no

---

[52] Ketogenic diet — It implies a severe restriction of carbohydrates, moderate use of healthy fats and proteins. It induces a Ketosis state: Benefits weight loss, improved insulin sensitivity, and increased mental clarity. It is recommended in certain forms of epilepsy and of hypersomnia. Risks - low blood pressure, nutrient deficiencies, constipation, increased risk of kidney and heart disorders.

[53] Paleo diet — implies the use of foods likely used by our Palaeolithic ancestors. It includes lean meats, fish, fruits, vegetables, nuts, and seeds while excluding grains, legumes, dairy products, and processed foods. Benefits: weight loss, improved blood sugar control, and better digestion. Risks: nutrients deficiency. Drawbacks: Restrictive food choices, costs, difficulty in restaurants, sustainability

[54] Intermittent fasting involves cycling between periods of fasting and eating; usually people skip breakfast and restrict their eating window to 8 hours, typically from noon to 8 pm. Benefits: weight loss, improved insulin sensitivity, and cellular repair processes. Risks: inability to support prolonged fasting (hypoglycaemia).

Sally – We both use routinely the Mediterranean diet, i.e, a diet rich in fruits, vegetables, whole grains, olive oil, fish, lean meat, eggs, moderate amounts of dairy products, and dry fruits. It includes moderate intake of red wine and limited consumption of red meat, processed foods, and sweets (occasionally is not a "crime").

Roger – The health benefits have been proven scientifically in many studies: a reduced risk of heart disease, lower blood pressure, improved cognitive function, better weight management, better physical and mental health and better compliance to COVID19[55]

From the lifestyles of this group some information concerning the connections between work and food habits can be found.

Processed foods and burgers mostly by some that work too much, gourmet recipes for those that are eventually too wealthy, heavier foods for those more linked to rural lifestyles, vegan for activists, and Mediterranean diet for other types of social activism.

It is very important that schoolteachers are acquainted with students eating, since many studies in many countries, from childhood to young adults, confirm their relationship with sleep, the relation between sleep duration and body mass index[56], and the relation with academic performance and quality of life[57]. An American study showed that skipping breakfast, late-night snacks, replacing meals with snacks, and irregular mealtimes

[55] Gaspar T, Paiva T, Matos MG Ecological model explaining the compliance to COVID-19, Int. J. Environ. Res. Public Health 2022, 19, 5159. https://doi.org/10.3390/ijerph19095159.

[56] Paiva T, Gaspar T, Matos MG Mutual relations between sleep deprivation, sleep stealers and risk behaviours in adolescents. Sleep Science 2016, Jan-Mar;9(1):7-13. http://dx.doi.org/10.1016/j.slsci.2016.02.176.

[57] Matos MG, Paiva T, Costa D, Gaspar T, Galvao D **Caffeine, Sleep Duration and Adolescents' Perception of Health Related Quality of Life.** British Journal of Education, Society & Behavioural Science 2016, 16(2):1-9.

were the best correlates with poor sleep quality[58]. *A Spanish study in school aged children showed that late sleep patterns, short sleep duration, and greater sleep disturbances are significantly related with what* and *how* school-aged children eat, *namely poor diet quality or irregular schedules*[59].

However, it must be said that often the relations are complex; they are found via a cluster of factors (eating habits, other habits, sleep, environment, behaviours) and its interference with important features of children/adolescents/young adults' life.

Furthermore, healthy lifestyles in adults, including eating habits, are crucial for prevention cardiovascular risk[60]. *The impact upon gastric adenocarcinoma is impressive*[61]; *the higher incidence was associated with poor sleep quality, smoking frequency, frying cooking habit, pickled food, thin liquid intake after meal, swallowing hot food without adequate cooling, doing other things while eating, eating overnight food, and eating midnight snack; while lower incidence was associated more frequently eating vegetables/fruit, beans, or kelps*

To sleep and live well, eat well

58 Faris ME, Vitiello MV, Abdelrahim DN, Cheikh Ismail L, Jahrami HA, Khaleel S, Khan MS, Shakir AZ, Yusuf AM, Masaad AA, Bahammam AS. Eating habits are associated with subjective sleep quality outcomes among university students: findings of a cross-sectional study. Sleep Breath. 2022 Sep;26(3):1365-1376. doi: 10.1007/s11325-021-02506-w. Epub 2021 Oct 6. PMID: 34613509.

59 Ramírez-Contreras C, Santamaría-Orleans A, Izquierdo-Pulido M, Zerón-Rugerio MF. Sleep dimensions are associated with obesity, poor diet quality and eating behaviors in school-aged children. Front Nutr. 2022 Sep 23;9:959503. doi: 10.3389/fnut.2022.959503. PMID: 36211495; PMCID: PMC9539562.

60 Kaminsky LA, German C, Imboden M, Ozemek C, Peterman JE, Brubaker PH. The importance of healthy lifestyle behaviors in the prevention of cardiovascular disease. Prog Cardiovasc Dis. 2022 Jan-Feb;70:8-15. doi: 10.1016/j.pcad.2021.12.001. Epub 2021 Dec 16. PMID: 34922952.

61 Huang L, Chen L, Gui ZX, Liu S, Wei ZJ, Xu AM. Preventable lifestyle and eating habits associated with gastric adenocarcinoma: A case-control study. J Cancer. 2020 Jan 1;11(5):1231-1239. doi: 10.7150/jca.39023. PMID: 31956369; PMCID: PMC6959061.

2. WALKING THE DOG

Mr Morgan - I feel much better since I walk my dog twice every day. I lost weight and I am better mood

Mrs Smith – Well my Bella does wake me up every day at 5am, to eat. She grasps the door and barks to waking me up. I can't sleep afterwards.

Mrs Miller – I don't like dogs. Cats are much smarter and independent. My cat sleeps with me, peacefully. I feel great with its company.

Mr Brown – I don't like pets. They are costly and introduce further worries and obligations in daily life

Mrs Thomas – You are an egocentric guy. I couldn't live without my cats, 7, all of them in my bed!

Mrs Miller – 7 seven in your bed?! Do you manage to sleep?

Mrs Thomas – Well, usually yes, but sometimes they fight. Cats have strict hierarchies which sometimes are questioned. These days I wake up, since they jump and snort.

Mr William – Are you not afraid that they hurt you? It seems dangerous...

Mrs Thomas – you might be wright, but they are my little kids...

Mr Morris – I don't like cats, they are too individualist. Recently my dog died, and I am still mourning him.

Mr Johnson – My dogs sleep outside in the garden. Sometimes is boring since they bark to strangers and other animals. They are good house guards, and we pay for it waking up in the middle of the night.

Mr Wilson – Well the weekends I go to our farm to get some contacts with nature. Walking in the forest is nice, but I wake quite early either with the rooster or later with the donkeys. After lunch I must take a nap to compensate for sleep deprivation. My wife enjoys the farm animals immensely; she likes to feed the chicken, to collect their eggs and to talk with the donkeys. She sits nearby and enters in a sort of meditation, she reurns renewed after a weekend at the farm.

Mrs Thomas – The difference from my cats' co-sleeping is that neither the rooster nor the donkey sleep in your bed!

Mr Wilson – Oh, no! certainly not!

Mr Scott – Well this is in a farm, but I leave in a high city building and I wake up every morning with pigeons around. We tried lots of anti-pigeon measures, without success I must say. They are persistent and look quite happy.

Mrs White – Well I have birds, canaries. I adore listing to their singing. They are my hobby

Mr George – I have fishes, beautiful colours, beautiful movements. They give me silence and peace. I stay there looking at them swimming softly and silently around.

Mrs Simpson – I bought a small white rabbit when my granddaughter was 1 year old. He is still there. He is very clean and a good company but does not sleep with me. He has his own bed!

The relations between humans and animals are longstanding. They started with Domestication, and were followed by Companionship, utilitarian use in Work, Transportation and War, in Nutrition and Clothing, in Entertainment and Exhibition, and more recently in Scientific studies, Police helpers, and Therapies. Animals have been used as Symbols, Examples and are the key characters of Fables.

With industrialization they are progressively less used in work, war and transportation but they gained a significant place as human companion

The health benefits of pet ownership have been studied for mental health and sleep. The effects might be positive but negative effects such as zoonotic infections, bites and falls, together with increased costs and reduced freedom, might occur and must be considered individually for each person.

A recent metanalysis concluded that Pet ownership does not seem to influence owners' mental health, but it does influence their physical activity[62].

A systematic review suggests that pets provide benefits to those with mental health conditions[63] with special reference to the homelessness[64].

Pet ownership may benefit community-dwelling older adults by providing companionship, giving a sense of purpose and meaning, reducing loneliness and increasing socialisation[65].

[62] Martins CF, Soares JP, Cortinhas A, Silva L, Cardoso L, Pires MA, Mota MP. Pet's influence on humans' daily physical activity and mental health: a meta-analysis. Front Public Health. 2023 May 30;11:1196199. doi: 10.3389/fpubh.2023.1196199. PMID: 37325330; PMCID: PMC10262044.

[63] Brooks HL, Rushton K, Lovell K, Bee P, Walker L, Grant L, Rogers A. The powerof support from companion animals for people living with mental health problems: a systematic review and narrative synthesis of the evidence. BMC Psychiatry. 2018 Feb 5;18(1):31. doi: 10.1186/s12888-018-1613-2. PMID: 29402247; PMCID: PMC5800290.

[64] Cleary M, West S, Visentin D, Phipps M, Westman M, Vesk K, Kornhaber R. The Unbreakable Bond: The Mental Health Benefits and Challenges of Pet Ownership for People Experiencing Homelessness. Issues Ment Health Nurs. 2021 Aug;42(8):741-746. doi: 10.1080/01612840.2020.1843096. Epub 2020 Nov 16. PMID:33196324.

[65] Hui Gan GZ, Hill AM, Yeung P, Keesing S, Netto JA. Pet ownership and its influence on mental health in older adults. Aging Ment Health. 2020 Oct;24(10):1605-1612. doi: 10.1080/13607863.2019.1633620. Epub 2019 Jun 27. PMID: 31242754.

Studies during COVID 19 showed negative effects of pet ownership pet ownership suggesting that during a specific situation such as a pandemic, pets may contribute to increased burden[66,67].

Pet death may be traumatic for children and associated with subsequent mental health difficulties[68]; idem for adults, some do not overcome it and refuse further experiences.

Besides ownership, it is important to evaluate co-sleeping with animals.

A recent study in USA, using a nationally representative sample, showed that co-sleeping with pets was associated with poorer perceived sleep quality and greater insomnia severity; this negative impact sleep was associated with dog ownership but not with cat ownership, was more pronounced when individuals own a greater number of pets, and not impacted by bondedness to pets[69].

[66] Bennetts SK, Crawford SB, Howell TJ, Burgemeister F, Chamberlain C, Burke K, Nicholson JM. Parent and child mental health during COVID-19 in Australia: The role of pet attachment. PLoS One. 2022 Jul 25;17(7):e0271687. doi: 10.1371/journal.pone.0271687. PMID: 35877660; PMCID: PMC9312405

[67] Phillipou A, Tan EJ, Toh WL, Van Rheenen TE, Meyer D, Neill E, Sumner PJ, Rossell SL. Pet ownership and mental health during COVID-19 lockdown. Aust Vet J. 2021 Oct;99(10):423-426. doi: 10.1111/avj.13102. Epub 2021 Jun 23. PMID: 34164809.

[68] Crawford KM, Zhu Y, Davis KA, Ernst S, Jacobsson K, Nishimi K, Smith ADAC, Dunn EC. The mental health effects of pet death during childhood: is it better to have loved and lost than never to have loved at all? Eur Child Adolesc Psychiatry. 2021 Oct;30(10):1547-1558. doi: 10.1007/s00787-020-01594-5. Epub2020 Sep 10. PMID: 32910227; PMCID: PMC7943653.

[69] Chin BN, Singh T, Carothers AS. Co-sleeping with pets, stress, and sleep in a nationally representative sample of United States adults. Sci Rep. 2024 Mar 6;14(1):5577. doi: 10.1038/s41598-024-56055-9. PMID: 38448628; PMCID: PMC10918166.

Preliminary results suggest that co-sleeping with a pet may not impact sleep quality in children[70] and in adolescents[71].

To have a pet may be positive for physical and mental health, but this conclusion is not universal and may be influenced by the owner characteristics, pet characteristics and environmental circumstances.

Co-sleeping may be OK, but it is not recommended with many animals, sick animals and animals with bad behaviours.

[70]   Rowe H, Jarrin DC, Noel NAO, Ramil J, McGrath JJ. The curious incident of the dog in the nighttime: The effects of pet-human co-sleeping and bedsharing on sleep dimensions of children and adolescents. Sleep Health. 2021 Jun;7(3):324-331. doi: 10.1016/j.sleh.2021.02.007. Epub 2021 Apr 30. PMID:33935015.
[71]   Rosano J, Howell T, Conduit R, Bennett P. Co-Sleeping between Adolescents and Their Pets May Not Impact Sleep Quality. Clocks Sleep. 2021 Jan 4;3(1):1-11. doi: 10.3390/clockssleep3010001. PMID: 33406702; PMCID: PMC7838871

3. HAVE A HOBBY, ENJOY NATURE, BE HAPPIER

Mr. Taylor – At present you know, I have nothing to do. I live alone, since I divorced some years ago, and my son and daughter are far away and busy with their own life. I visit them once or twice a year. Traveling is expensive and tiring.

Doctor – Well, Mr Taylor, which are your daily routines?

Mr. Taylor – I wake quite early, around 5 or 6 am, and then breakfast, TV news, I go to Starbucks, 2nd breakfast, I sit there, see people around, newspaper, go home, eat something, nap, TV series, domestic cleaning, dinner, reading, TV, bed.

Doctor – Well, Mr Taylor, do you sleep well?

Mr. Taylor – No, despite medication I have great difficulty falling asleep and wake up several times.

Doctor – Do you eat well?

Mr. Taylor – Not really, I would say. No patience to cook, so .... many processed foods

Doctor – Do you walk or exercise? Are you outside, in the open air?

Mr. Taylor – Not really, I would say.

Doctor – You will never sleep well with your present habits. Let's see what you would like to do. What about music, dancing, singing, drawing, painting, photography, meditation, reading, crafts with ceramics, wood, stone etc, home repairs, gardening, cooking, discussion groups, museums, crosswords/sudoku, puzzles, collections ...?

Mr. Taylor – Well! I have never done nothing of the kind! Can you repeat it

Doctor – OK I will say it again, but it is quite important that you keep your brain, your hands, and your body busy with pleasant activities to be healthier, happier and sleep. Furthermore, you must be outside in the open air, to get sun light and fresh air. You must exercise and eat well. Finally, you must socialize, to be and talk with other people, to share things, discuss subjects of interest and laugh. At present you are doing nothing of this, so your physical and mental health can't be good.

Mr. Taylor – Indeed ... you are right

Doctor – Ok let's start with the hobbies.

- Music: you can listen to music, go to concerts, learn to play an instrument (piano, guitar, drums...)
- Dancing: you can go to a dancing school and learn classic (Tango, Walz, ..) or modern dances (Hip hop, Zumba, ...)
- Singing: you can have lessons, join a choir, practice karaoke
- Drawing, painting, photography: you can have lessons, join groups, make a course, try for yourself
- Meditation, yoga, Tai-chi, other: you can have lessons, join groups, make a course
- Reading: it is very good but, it is a lonely act, and when we are older feedback is important, so I would advise reading clubs or book discussion with friends
- Crafts with ceramics, wood, stone, needle, textiles, paper, natural products (leaves, shells, flowers, ...) etc,
- Home repairs and do it yourself: it is for you to choose what to do
- Cooking, making jams or liquors – you can learn how to cook for yourself and how to eat healthy, make courses, buy books, join groups
- Discussion groups – they promote socialization; take care with "toxic" people
- Museums, exhibitions – go and visit, join a group

- Crosswords, sudoku, solitaires, card games, other games — alone you train cognition and memory, with others you amuse yourself and train strategies
- Puzzles 2D or 3D - train cognition, vision, memory, fine hand movements, spatial memory
- Collections of whatever, millions of choices, a good entertainment not necessarily expensive

Doctor — Is this enough? Do you still need more choices?

Mr. Taylor — Thanks for the explanation. I will think about it, if you don't mind

Doctor — Well I would like to explain to you some hobbies that include exercise and nature connectedness

- Walking and hiking — Our ancestors went from Afrika to Europe and Asia mainly walking. So, walking around near gardens, ponds, rivers or the seacoast is fantastic. Idem for hiking in wilder environments; better do not go alone.
- Gardening, floriculture, vegetables, fruit, microgreens, hydroponics, etc: you can learn, you can study, you can try, you can join groups
- Forest bathes are quite therapeutic: join groups, better do not go alone.

Mr. Taylor — You are convincing me. I will come back with good news.

Hobbies are in principle related to neurological functioning and can be divided according to their main function: 1) Inducing pleasure; 2) Brain reward system activation; 3) Relaxation promotion; 4) Cognitive function preservation[72].

Music, dancing, singing, drawing, painting, photography, meditation, reading, arts and crafts, home repairs, gardening,

---

[72] Gutman SA, Schindler VP. The neurological basis of occupation. Occup Ther Int. 2007;14(2):71-85. doi: 10.1002/oti.225. PMID: 17623380.

cooking, etc, can stimulate the neurological system and enhance health and well-being.

The sedation and activation effects of music are known for centuries, with special music to precede battles, football and Olympic games and lullabies for babies. In the context of this chapter music can be a hobby or a therapy to induce sleep. As a hobby music improves mental health, however, despite many studies using music therapy for sleep, poor methodologic issues prevent generalizations; clear results have been obtained in paediatric populations[73] and with project Sleep[74].

In a multinational evaluation of more than 90000 old adults, having a hobby was associated with fewer depressive symptoms, higher levels of self-reported health, happiness and life satisfaction[75].

In teachers, hobbies improve emotional well-being and coping stress strategies[76].

For medical students in USA ten clusters of self-care activities were identified: nourishment, hygiene, intellectual and creative health, physical activity, spiritual care, balance and relaxation,

[73] Loewy J. Music Therapy as a Potential Intervention for Sleep Improvement. Nat Sci Sleep. 2020 Jan 7;12:1-9. doi: 10.2147/NSS.S194938. PMID: 32021519; PMCID: PMC6954684.

[74] Chang-Lit W, Loewy J, Fox J, Grabscheid E, Fogel J. Project sleep: the role and effect of a comprehensive, multidisciplinary music therapy quality improvement program. J Sleep Dis Res. 2018;1 (2):26–41. doi:10.14302/issn.2574-4518. jsdr-17-1785

[75] Mak HW, Noguchi T, Bone JK, Wels J, Gao Q, Kondo K, Saito T, Fancourt D. Hobby engagement and mental wellbeing among people aged 65 years and older in 16 countries. Nat Med. 2023 Sep;29(9):2233-2240. doi: 10.1038/s41591-023-02506-1. Epub 2023 Sep 11. PMID: 37696932; PMCID: PMC10504079.

[76] Emeljanovas A, Sabaliauskas S, Mežienė B, Istomina N. The relationships between teachers' emotional health and stress coping. Front Psychol. 2023 Nov 20;14:1276431. doi: 10.3389/fpsyg.2023.1276431. PMID: 38054175; PMCID: PMC10694432.

time for loved ones, big picture goals, pleasure and outside activities, and hobbies[77].

An international survey in 87 different countries involving mostly women between 41 to 60 years showed that crochet offers positive benefits for personal wellbeing with many respondents actively using crochet to manage mental health conditions and life events such as grief, chronic illness and pain[78]; these results were also proven for all sorts of needle crafting (sewing, crocheting, knitting, lacemaking, embroidery and quilting) in a recent review[79].

Results from the HEartS Survey in UK showed that over 97% of respondents reported engagement in one or more arts activities at least once during 2018-2019, with reading and listening to music being the most popular activities; more arts engagement was associated with higher levels of wellbeing, social connectedness, and lower odds of intense social loneliness, however in excessive consumption there was a positive association with depression and intense emotional loneliness[80].

During COVID 19 Increased time spent gardening was associated with reductions in depressive and anxiety symptoms and enhanced

[77]   Ayala EE, Omorodion AM, Nmecha D, Winseman JS, Mason HRC. What Do Medical Students Do for Self-Care? A Student-Centered Approach to Well-Being. Teach Learn Med. 2017 Jul-Sep;29(3):237-246. doi: 10.1080/10401334.2016.1271334. Epub2017 Feb 16. PMID: 28632007.

[78]   Burns P, Van Der Meer R. Happy Hookers: findings from an international study exploring the effects of crochet on wellbeing. Perspect Public Health. 2021 May;141(3):149-157. doi: 10.1177/1757913920911961. Epub 2020 Apr 3. PMID: 32245337.

[79]   Le Lagadec D, Kornhaber R, Johnston-Devin C, Cleary M. Healing Stitches: AScoping Review on the Impact of Needlecraft on Mental Health and Well-Being. Issues Ment Health Nurs. 2024 Jul 15:1-14. doi: 10.1080/01612840.2024.2364228. Epub ahead of print. PMID: 39008815.

[80]   Tymoszuk U, Spiro N, Perkins R, Mason-Bertrand A, Gee K, Williamon A. Arts engagement trends in the United Kingdom and their mental and social wellbeing implications: HEartS Survey. PLoS One. 2021 Mar 12;16(3):e0246078. doi: 10.1371/journal.pone.0246078. PMID: 33711028; PMCID: PMC7954337.

life satisfaction and spending more time doing woodwork/DIY and arts/crafts were also associated with enhanced life satisfaction[81].

Multiple linear regression indicated that maintaining or increasing time on leisure activities significantly predicted well-being during COVID-19, with increased time spent on home crafts and artisanship, fine arts, musical and performing arts engagement, sports and outdoor pursuits, niche and IT interests, and language activities each predicting higher well-being outcomes[82].

In a cross-cultural study in India and Canada laughter was associated with emotional well-being in Canada and life satisfaction in India[83]. Humour orientation was associated with increased mental well-being, lower levels of loneliness, and less headaches in young adults[84].

Yoga as monotherapy or adjunctive therapy shows positive effects for depression. As an adjunctive therapy, it facilitates treatment of anxiety disorders. Tai chi and qi gong may be helpful as adjunctive therapies for depression, but effects are inconsistent.

---

[81] Bone JK, Fancourt D, Sonke JK, Fluharty ME, Cohen R, Lee JB, Kolenic AJ, Radunovich H, Bu F. Creative leisure activities, mental health and well-being during 5 months of the COVID-19 pandemic: a fixed effects analysis of data from 3725 US adults. J Epidemiol Community Health. 2023 May;77(5):293-297. doi: 10.1136/jech-2022-219653. Epub 2023 Feb 27. PMID: 36849241; PMCID: PMC10086468

[82] Morse KF, Fine PA, Friedlander KJ. Creativity and Leisure During COVID-19: Examining the Relationship Between Leisure Activities, Motivations, and Psychological Well-Being. Front Psychol. 2021 Jul 5;12:609967. doi: 10.3389/fpsyg.2021.609967. PMID: 34290635; PMCID: PMC8288551.

[83] Hasan H, Hasan TF. Laugh yourself into a healthier person: a cross cultural analysis of the effects of varying levels of laughter on health. Int J Med Sci. 2009 Jul 28;6(4):200-11. doi: 10.7150/ijms.6.200. PMID: 19652724; PMCID: PMC2719285

[84] Curran T, Janovec A, Olsen K. Making Others Laugh is the Best Medicine: Humor Orientation, Health Outcomes, and the Moderating Role of Cognitive Flexibility. Health Commun. 2021 Apr;36(4):468-475. doi: 10.1080/10410236.2019.1700438. Epub 2019 Dec 10. PMID: 31818148

As monotherapy or an adjunctive therapy, mindfulness-based meditation has positive effects on depression[85].

Nature therapy as a health-promotion method is implicated for the reduction of reported modern-day "stress-state" and "technostress"[86]. Evidence suggests beneficial therapeutic effects of forest-based interventions on hypertension, stress, and mental-health disorders, such as depression and anxiety[87]. The effects are, at least in part, associated with lowering cortisol levels; a meta-analysis showed that salivary cortisol levels were significantly lower in the forest groups compared with the urban groups[88].

A meta-analysis, including papers from USA, Europe, Asia and Middle East showed that gardening has positive association with health outcomes, such as reductions in depression and anxiety symptoms, stress, mood disturbance, and BMI, it increases quality of life, sense of community, physical activity levels, and cognitive function[89].

---

[85] Saeed SA, Cunningham K, Bloch RM. Depression and Anxiety Disorders: Benefits of Exercise, Yoga, and Meditation. Am Fam Physician. 2019 May 15;99(10):620-627.PMID: 31083878

[86] Hansen MM, Jones R, Tocchini K. Shinrin-Yoku (Forest Bathing) and Nature Therapy: A State-of-the-Art Review. Int J Environ Res Public Health. 2017 Jul 28;14(8):851. doi: 10.3390/ijerph14080851. PMID: 28788101; PMCID: PMC5580555.

[87] Stier-Jarmer M, Throner V, Kirschneck M, Immich G, Frisch D, Schuh A. The Psychological and Physical Effects of Forests on Human Health: A Systematic Review of Systematic Reviews and Meta-Analyses. Int J Environ Res Public Health. 2021 Feb 11;18(4):1770. doi: 10.3390/ijerph18041770. PMID: 33670337; PMCID: PMC7918603.

[88] Antonelli M, Barbieri G, Donelli D. Effects of forest bathing (shinrin-yoku) on levels of cortisol as a stress biomarker: a systematic review and meta-analysis. Int J Biometeorol. 2019 Aug;63(8):1117-1134. doi:10.1007/s00484-019-01717-x. Epub 2019 Apr 18. PMID: 31001682.1. Int J Environ Res Public Health. 2021 Feb 11;18(4):1770. doi: 10.3390/ijerph18041770.

[89] Soga M, Gaston KJ, Yamaura Y. Gardening is beneficial for health: A meta-analysis. Prev Med Rep. 2016 Nov 14;5:92-99. doi: 10.1016/j.pmedr.2016.11.007. PMID: 27981022; PMCID: PMC5153451.

In synthesis:

Pleasure and occupational hedonic activities have positive aspects upon health and wellbeing

Open air activities and connectedness with Nature improve your quality of life

4. MY DAILY SCHEDULES ARE WELL ORGANIZED

Jane – You are late today

Jamie – I'm sorry. I could not find my mobile and yesterday I went late to bed. My wife chose an old movie, and we could not stop seeing it

Jane - Which one?

Jamie – "Gone with the Wind". Have you seen it?

Jane – No! We must hurry now, otherwise we will be late

Jamie – OK Mrs Punctuality. Let's go

Jane – I live with my watch. Waking up at 6:22 am, Gym at 6:30, Shower at 7:00, Dressing at 7:15, Breakfast at 7:35, Ready 7:50

Jamie - Wow!! If someday you have children, these minutes and regularities disappear.

Jane – That's the reason I don't want children. I can't live in a mess.

Jamie – At what time do you eat and go to bed

Jane – Lunch at 12:00, Five o Clock tea is at 4:30pm, Out of work at 6:40, Dinner at 7:30pm, Tv and shower, Bed routines at 9:45, in bed at 10pm, podcast, lights out 10:15.

Jamie - Do you sleep well?

Jane – Well... I have some difficulties ...

They were approaching work. Jamie looks attentively at Jane. Everything in her was in order and perfect: the haircut, the makeup, the white blouse, the brown skirt, but ... around the eyes small black circles were silently emerging ...

Jane was not happy and did not sleep well — he thought. But Jane also wanted answers ...

Jane — And what about you and your schedules?

Jamie — Well, Jane, I am not so organized. I wake up between 6:45/7:15, Start working around 8/8:15, have my morning coffee around 10 /10:30, have lunch between 12:30 /1pm; Out of work at 5pm. Pick up children from school and confusion starts... Dinner depends on who is making it. Children SSB, ie, Shower/Shouting/Bed. Exhausted at TV for news and movie. Mary falls asleep in sofa. Carrying Mary to bed and sleep

Jane — Quite tiring!

Jamie — Yes, but warm and recomforting. Mary is quite disorganized; she is never on time! Never wakes up at the desirable time, is late for work, for meals, for bed for everything. She sleeps several times a day, saying she is doing as Da Vinci. The great Leonard had a polyphasic sleep. She gets nervous when I press her.

The 3 daily routine schedules of Jane, Jamie and Mary are quite different

Jane is certainly perfectionist and too much organized: everything is settled at the range of minutes-

Jamie adapts to the work and family life the best he can

Mary has no proper schedules and no daily routine despite the so called polyphasic sleep[90].

---

[90] Weaver MD, Sletten TL, Foster RG, Gozal D, Klerman EB, Rajaratnam SMW, Roenneberg T, Takahashi JS, Turek FW, Vitiello MV, Young MW, Czeisler CA. Adverse impact of polyphasic sleep patterns in humans: Report of the National Sleep Foundation sleep timing and variability consensus panel. Sleep Health. 2021 Jun;7(3):293-302. doi: 10.1016/j.sleh.2021.02.009. Epub 2021 Mar 29. PMID: 33795195.

It is important to have daily routines and regular sleep schedules, but our body and our sleep are not metronomes and everything in our physiology is adaptive within certain limits. So Jamie daily routines are more beneficial for his own health, Jane risk to develop insomnia and Mary with poor routines and a disorganized polyphasic sleep also faces troubles both in her sleep and her health.

5. I LYE ON BED ALL DAY

Mrs Emma enters the room, looks around, moves slowly and sits down looking at me. A friend, a bit younger, is coming with her. Looking seriously to me she tells her story

— I am old now, 76 next month and ... I don't sleep for years, many years. As I don't sleep well I can't do nothing properly. I live alone, you know. I always took care of my house and my things and nowadays I do almost nothing. As I don't sleep at night I go to bed trying to sleep or rest. My Pussy goes with me, and we are in bed all day long. Pussy is quite nice, white, green eyes, a black spot around the nose. My company. For him I do something, preparing his food, fresh water, cleaning ... For me I do the least possible, eat bread, can food, things easy to do.

She looks pale and tired, while pointing to her friend

— My friend brings me soup and fruit several times a week. She tries to take me out of home, but I am too tired since I don't sleep

Mrs Olivia, Emma's friend, got agitated

— I am always telling her that she must go out and can't be lying on bed all day long. She was very active in older days. We travelled a lot, went to parties, theatres and concerts, but now .... She and the cat always in bed.

It was time to clarify symptoms objectively

— How many hours per day are you lying in bed? At what time do you wake?
— I wake quite early, but I get out of bed around 10am, drink a glass of milk, do something around but at 11 or 12am I go

to bed again since I am tired. Eat some cookies and try to sleep until 3 or 4pm. Then I see a soap opera that I like at 4. At 7pm I eat something and as it dark and cold I go to bed again around 8pm, in order to sleep and be warmer. Then I don't sleep, and the night goes on and on... Medications do nothing I tried many already. I count the hours of the church bell, so I know I am awake. Hera is a paper with all the medications so far... It's a curse, Doctor, it's a curse!

It was better to change subject

— Well, you are in bed around 16 to 17 hours per day, you don't eat properly, you don't move, we do almost nothing, you are alone with Pussy and don't socialize. Of course, you don't sleep and you will not sleep if you go on doing the same.
— I am like that because I don't sleep!!!
— I do not agree with you, but I will explain everything latter. Did you make any blood tests, sleep tests, whatever?
— I made a sleep teste at home. They say I slept 6 hours. It is impossible. I know that I was awake all night.
— Ok let's see.

Mrs Emma's case has multiple aspects.

Her sleep complaint of not sleeping is contradicted by the Polysomnography result stating that she slept 6hours, value relatively normal for her age.

This contradiction suggests a diagnosis no longer in use of Paradoxical Insomnia[91,92], that is, a severe insomnia subjective

[91] Rezaie L, Fobian AD, McCall WV, Khazaie H. Paradoxical insomnia and subjective-objective sleep discrepancy: A review. Sleep Med Rev. 2018 Aug; 40:196-202. doi: 10.1016/j.smrv.2018.01.002. Epub 2018 Jan 6. PMID: 29402512.
[92] Castelnovo A, Ferri R, Punjabi NM, Castronovo V, Garbazza C, Zucconi M, Ferini-Strambi L, Manconi M. The paradox of paradoxical insomnia: A theoretical review towards a unifying evidence-based definition. Sleep Med Rev. 2019 Apr;44:70-82. doi: 10.1016/j.smrv.2018.12.007. Epub 2018 Dec 25. PMID: 30731262.

complaint not objectively confirmed with marked discrepancy between both, as described in the ICSD2[93]. It must be said that this subjective misperception of sleep as wakefulness, which impacts upon the subjective evaluation of sleep duration, is not specific of paradoxical insomnia and can occur in other disorders.

The other important aspect is the prolonged time in bed, which has the same serious health risks of sleep deprivation and sleep extension.

Besides that, she does not go out, she does not get sun light, she does not eat properly, makes no exercise, has no objectives beyond treating the cat, feels quite lonely[94] and is a bit stubborn.

Altogether all these facts are very dangerous for an elderly person, and require efficient treatment

Treatment pointed for each of them: 1) Sleep misperception – attempt to convince her by explaining and showing the polysomnography data that she slept something; 2) Reducing drastically the time in bed and implementing daily routines; 3) Asking her friend, Mrs Olivia, support for adequate nutrition and going out; 4) Managing rationally her medication; 5) Asking blood tests to identify and correct possible deficits or abnormalities; 6) Suggestion if interests, activities and socialization to overcome loneliness.

It took time, but nowadays it is very rewarding to see her smiling and laughing, and saying she sleeps enough

Too much time in bed is a poison

No sun light is terrible

---

[93] ICSD2 – International Classification of Sleep Disorders, published in 2005, and discarded in the new classification ICSD3

[94] Paiva T, Gaspar T, Tomé G, Matos, MG. Loneliness during the COVID pandemic: characteristics and associated risks. MOJ Public Health. 2024;13(2):131-140. DOI: 10.15406/mojph.2024.13.00451

6. I DON'T LIKE GYMS

In my family everybody likes sports, except myself.

My husband disappears during the weekends to play golf

My oldest son, William, plays tennis semi-professionally. He plays during the week the early morning and weekends all day

My daughter, Rita, is a swimmer and is preparing for the National championship. She trains every weekday from 9 to 10:30 pm

My younger daughter, Margaret, practise rhythmic gym. She trains three times a week from 8 to 9:30 pm

The youngest, Robert, is a football player. He trains two times a week from 8 to 9:30pm

My self I practise gym sited at the sofa and doing nothing, except TV watching

Physical activity is, together with nutrition and sleep a fundamental pillar of Health

However, care must be taken whenever analysing or practicing physical activity.

No physical activity and sitting for long periods are terrible, both for health and for sleep, as it has been proven in systematic reviews[95] and in a large population sample during COVID; poor physical activity is associated with poor mental and physical health and

---

[95] De Nys L, Anderson K, Ofosu EF, Ryde GC, Connelly J, Whittaker AC. The effects of physical activity on cortisol and sleep: A systematic review and meta-analysis. Psychoneuroendocrinology. 2022 Sep;143:105843. doi: 10.1016/j.psyneuen.2022.105843. Epub 2022 Jun 24. PMID: 35777076.

worse compliance with COVOD constraints[96]. This is the mother situation! Take care and start moving!

The father practise Golf, an open-air sport, with long walks and pauses. The COVID study showed that practice of physical activity between 4 and 10 hours per week was the best option. The father seems to fit in: Congratulations!

The oldest son, William, plays tennis almost every day, at very early hours during the week and during many hours during weekends. It is an open-air sport which is very good, but he must take care not to curtail sleep during the week and not exaggerating in playing hours during the weekend. If not, Congratulations and don't forget that top tennis players sleep between 8 to 12hours a day!

The three younger brothers all train at night in indoor or outdoor spaces with intense lighting (swimming pools, gymnasiums and football fields). Intense light at night blocks melatonin production, furthermore, intense physical activity at night delays sleep onset. This means that both effects together will have a negative impact upon sleep. For Rita, Margaret and Robert I say: Good! but take care and try to practise at earlier hours.

For Margaret I also say that she must take care with diets and weight control and eat well, since exhaustion depression and sleepiness might occur if you exaggerate with your beautiful figure[97].

[96] Gaspar T, Paiva T, Matos MG Ecological model explaining the compliance to COVID-19, Int. J. Environ. Res. Public Health 2022, 19, 5159. https://doi.org/10.3390/ijerph19095159.

[97] Silva MR, Paiva T. Risk factors for precompetitive sleep behavior in elite female athletes The Journal of Sports Medicine and Physical Fitness 2019 April;59(4):708-16

7. THE BRAVE NEW WORLD: SCREENS AND INTERNET

It is a special dinner family in a beautiful restaurant at the seacoast, with a magnificent view.

They are many, two families together with three generations

After arrival and small talks and gossips they sit

Before the starters John, Mary and Rudy in their teens, start talking via the mobiles and laughing

Richard, a schoolboy, is playing a game attentively.

Little Sara, a toddler, has also a mobile and is playing with it.

Charlote is talking with Elizabeth, but both look regularly to the massages in their phones; their husbands do the same, both read the messages and receive phone calls, which they attend raising from table and going a bit apart

Grandma Brown and Granpa Smith look at each other and whisper. Dinners with everybody talking and laughing around the table belong to a distant past.

In the past decades technological development and internet had marked impact and improvement in Citizens and Societies life, changing positively all fields from habits, education and health to business, finance and politics.

Improvements are however associated with some dangers, which knowledge is critical to prevent and reduce them.

How Screen time affects Sleep, and which are the harms?

– *An increase of screen timing leads to mismanagement of time, leading to less sleeping time[98];*

– *The contents of media may cause physiological/ psychological excitement, interfering with the ability to fall asleep[98];*

– *The light emitted from screens affects the circadian system and causes alertness[99]*

– *In all ages excessive use of technology reduces sleep duration and sleep efficiency with increased awakenings; it also promotes late bedtimes*

– *The sedentary, indoors screen use, reduces exposure to sun light, which further affects sleep and promotes late bedtimes*

Which are the harms of excessive screens to our bodies?

– *Musculoskeletal discomfort, mostly in the neck, lower back and shoulders, and forward head posture are quite frequent, mainly in adolescents, in mobile phone or tablets users*

– *Ophthalmologic problems include dry eye, increased myopia prevalence and eye fatigue*

– *Muscular tension increases with possible association with headaches and tendinitis*

– *Sedentarism with increased risk of excessive weight and cardiovascular problems*

– *Fatigue*

---

[98] Anderson CA, Bushman BJ. Effects of violent video games on aggressive behavior, aggressive cognition, aggressive affect, physiological arousal, and prosocial behavior: a meta-analytic review of the scientific literature. Psychol Sci. 2001 Sep;12(5):353-9. doi: 10.1111/1467-9280.00366. PMID: 11554666.

[99] Higuchi S, Motohashi Y, Liu Y, Maeda A. Effects of playing a computer game using a bright display on presleep physiological variables, sleep latency, slow wave sleep and REM sleep. J Sleep Res. 2005 Sep;14(3):267-73. doi: 10.1111/j.1365-2869.2005.00463.x. PMID: 16120101.

Which are the potential harms of excessive technology use to our brains[100]?

- *Reduced attention – with increased symptoms of ADHD in children and adolescents and attention deficits in people of all ages. The mechanisms related to attention difficulties are related with the repetitive attentional shifts and multitasking, which can impair executive functioning. Constant technology use prevents the brain to rest in its default mode.*
- *Impaired emotional and social intelligence due to reduced physical contact*
- *Internet addiction – addicted children have greater symptoms of inattention, hyperactivity, and impulsivity. In adults' addiction predictors are younger age, playing massively multiplayer online role-playing games, and spending more time online.*
- *Social isolation – use of social media more than 2 hours per day increases the rate of social isolation in young, middle-aged and older adults*
- *Cognitive and brain development – small children using screens have poorer language development; in pre-adolescent children more screen and less reading time were associated with decreased brain connectivity between regions controlling word recognition and cognitive control.*

Which are the potential harms of excessive technology use and social networks involvement to Behaviour and Mental health?

---

[100] Small GW, Lee J, Kaufman A, Jalil J, Siddarth P, Gaddipati H, Moody TD, Bookheimer SY. Brain health consequences of digital technology use. Dialogues Clin Neurosci. 2020 Jun;22(2):179-187. doi: 10.31887/DCNS.2020.22.2/gsmall. PMID: 32699518; PMCID: PMC7366948.

- *Risk behaviours in adolescents (alcohol, drugs and tobacco consumption, violence, premature and unprotected sex[101]. Higher prevalence of new-onset disruptive behaviour disorders (conduct disorder and oppositional defiant disorder)[102].*
- *Violence and violence promotion in adults – physical, sexual, gun violence perpetration and violent protests are fostered in specific social networks. Factors often associated with violence are the desperate search for popularity, the sense of protection of anonymity, a violent environment. Factors associated with victimization are low self-esteem, loneliness and low protection from adults.*
- *Depression, anxiety, loneliness[103]*
- *Sexuality -* **Sexting is spreading dangerously among adolescents who share private and explicit sexual content, ignoring the associated negative and risky consequences[104] The odds of ever having sex was 31% higher among those with high TV usage, 43% higher among those with high recreational computer usage, and 54% higher among**

[101] Paiva T, Gaspar T, Matos MG. Mutual relations between sleep deprivation, sleep stealers and risk behaviours in adolescents. Sleep Sci. 2016 Jan-Mar;9(1):7-13. doi: 10.1016/j.slsci.2016.02.176. Epub 2016 Feb 23. PMID: 27226817; PMCID: PMC4867935.

[102] Nagata JM, Chu J, Ganson KT, Murray SB, Iyer P, Gabriel KP, Garber AK, Bibbins-Domingo K, Baker FC. Contemporary screen time modalities and disruptive behavior disorders in children: a prospective cohort study. J Child Psychol Psychiatry. 2023 Jan;64(1):125-135. doi: 10.1111/jcpp.13673. Epub 2022 Jul 26. PMID: 35881083; PMCID: PMC9771898.

[103] Twenge JM, Campbell WK. Associations between screen time and lower psychological well-being among children and adolescents: Evidence from a population-based study. Prev Med Rep. 2018 Oct 18;12:271-283. doi: 10.1016/j.pmedr.2018.10.003. PMID: 30406005; PMCID: PMC6214874.

[104] Verrastro V, Saladino V, Eleuteri S, Barberis N, Cuzzocrea F. Sexting, Self-esteem, and Social Media: A Comparison among Frequent, Occasional, and Non-sexting Italian Adolescent Girls. Psychol Russ. 2023 Dec 1;16(4):3-20. doi:10.11621/pir.2023.0401. PMID: 38162809; PMCID: PMC10755954.

those with extremely high (6+ hours) total screen time[105]. The use of social networks by sexual minorities reduces loneliness[106]. Sexual minority adolescents reported more screen time and higher problematic screen use than heterosexual peers[107].

Potential benefits of technologies for elders

- Searching online may be a form of brain neural exercise, which may benefit brain health and delay cognitive decline
- Short-term internet-search training may increase white-matter integrity in the right superior longitudinal fasciculus, which could result from increased myelination[108].
- Computerized cognitive training has an overall moderate effect on cognition in mild cognitive impairment. Small to moderate effects were reported for global cognition, attention, working memory, and learning abilities.

---

[105] Barr EM, Moore MJ, Johnson T, Merten J, Stewart WP The Relationship between Screen Time and Sexual Behaviors among Middle School Students. *Health Educator*, v46 n1 p6-13 Spr 2014

[106] Charmaraman L, Zhang A, Wang K, Chen B. Sexual Minorities and Loneliness: Exploring Sexuality through Social Media and Gender-Sexuality Alliance (GSA) Supports. Int J Environ Res Public Health. 2024 Mar 4;21(3):300. doi:10.3390/ijerph21030300. PMID: 38541299; PMCID: PMC10970596.

[107] Nagata JM, Lee CM, Yang J, Al-Shoaibi AAA, Ganson KT, Testa A, Jackson DB. Associations between sexual orientation and early adolescent screen use: findings from the Adolescent Brain Cognitive Development (ABCD) Study. Ann Epidemiol. 2023 Jun;82:54-58.e1. doi: 10.1016/j.annepidem.2023.03.004. Epub 2023 Mar 23. PMID: 36965838; PMCID: PMC10793659.

[108] Dong G, Hui L, Potenza MN. Short-term Internet-search training is associated with increased fractional anisotropy in the superior longitudinal fasciculus in the parietal lobe. *Front Neurosci*. 2017;11:372. doi: 10.3389/fnins.2017.00372.

8. RUINING SLEEP

"I haven't slept for about 6 months and stay awake all night. I don't have any serious problems, and life is fine, but I just cannot sleep."

"Do you drink a lot of coffee?"

"Of course, I do. Coffee helps me sleep better. I always have one at the end of a meal and one more before going to bed. It surely can't be that. I have been doing that for years and always slept well."

"Hmm! And do you drink alcohol?"

"Not during lunch, but at dinner I have two or three glasses to help the food go down."

"Anything else?"

"Well then I sit down and have a generous whisky with ice to help me relax."

"Just one?"

"Well sometimes two. They say that whisky is good for the circulation and helps avoid heart attacks."

"And do you drink anything else?"

"Coca-Cola. Just at lunch, one or two cans of Coca-Cola light to do less harm."

"Hmm! And do you eat well at dinner?"

"Of course, I do. I spend the day without eating so I devour my dinner. My wife cooks fantastically and I have to do the honours at home."

"And do you work out?"

"What does that mean? Gymnastics? God forbid. Who's got time? I spend the day stuck at a desk getting work done and at night I am so tired that I just eat, watch a little TV and go to bed."

"Do you actually watch or just fall asleep in front of the television?"

"Of course, I sleep! I sit down and boom! … and frankly it is always the same thing and not that good."

"And at weekends?"

"I have a few hearty lunches with my friends."

"So do you drink even more?"

"Yes of course. Those rich foods need to be eaten with wine and a coffee with a little milk helps to round it all off. Then I have a little nap. It's wonderful."

"Do you smoke?"

"Me?! Doctor, who doesn't smoke? Of course, I do, since I was 13 when I started to smoke to show I was a real man."

"How many cigarettes a day?"

"Let's see… a packet and a half, two packets."

"How much do you weigh?"

"The missus nags, but I weigh around 210 pounds (95 kg). It's her fault – she cooks so well."

"I am sorry to tell you, but you are behaving unwisely and putting your health at risk. Either you change your habits, or you risk getting several illnesses."

Sleep has its own hygiene which cannot be neglected.

In this case there are several harmful habits.

Coffee: *Sensitivity to caffeine is variable. Some people only feel the consequences from a certain age onwards, but caffeine produces insomnia because it links to the receptors for adenosine, increasing their numbers and so adenosine persists, and this makes sleep difficult, since it impacts upon sleep pressure. Caffeine consumption reduces 45 min in total sleep time and 7% of sleep efficiency, increases sleep onset latency by 9 min and wake after sleep onset by 12 min; the duration and relative proportion of light sleep increased while and the duration and relative proportion of deep sleep decreased[109]. Caffeine is present in coffee, in Coca-Cola, in tea and in many caffeinated drinks. Cutoff caffeine timing should be adjusted individually, the closer to bedtime the higher the effect.*

Alcohol: *alcohol facilitates falling asleep but makes sleep lighter, increasing light sleep and reducing REM sleep with increasing awakenings. It also impacts the circadian regulation blunting the overall normal diurnal variation in core body temperature rhythm and decreasing salivary melatonin levels[110]. Furthermore, it reduces or inhibits the breathing reflexes and reduces the tone of the respiratory muscles. Overall, these actions facilitate apnoeas; patients who snore or who have apnoeas should not drink alcohol at dinner time, or after it. People who suffer from periodic limb movements are also affected by the ingestion of alcohol. Insomniacs, afraid of medication, may try alcoholic beverages to induce sleep; this is quite wrong since alcohol will provoke a lighter sleep with increased awakenings; a real danger of alcohol dependence exists due to the need of dose increase.*

---

[109] Gardiner C, Weakley J, Burke LM, Roach GD, Sargent C, Maniar N, Townshend A, Halson SL. The effect of caffeine on subsequent sleep: A systematic review and meta-analysis. Sleep Med Rev. 2023 Jun;69:101764. doi: 10.1016/j.smrv.2023.101764. Epub 2023 Feb 6. PMID: 36870101.

[110] He S, Hasler BP, Chakravorty S. Alcohol and sleep-related problems. Curr Opin Psychol. 2019 Dec;30:117-122. doi: 10.1016/j.copsyc.2019.03.007. Epub 2019 Apr 19. PMID: 31128400; PMCID: PMC6801009.

Heavy meals at night make sleep more difficult and lighter[111]. *You should have regular meals throughout the day, more so at the start of the day and lighter towards the end of the day. You should not eat 2 hours prior to sleep.*

Light exposure at the evening and night blocks melatonin production and stimulates awakening; this might occur in those who use screens at late schedules, in sports practise in the evening in highly lighted environments (swimming pools, gyms, lighted open air camps, etc), in shift work, and late parties.

Tobacco: You should avoid tobacco; in excess it acts as a stimulant. It is important not to forget the negative effects of tobacco on the cardiovascular system, or the added risks of getting cancer. Furthermore, there is emerging evidence implicating tobacco smoking as a causal factor in onset of both common and severe mental illness[112]*; in line with this tobacco may impact sleep via a vicious circle, i.e., inducing both insomnia and a mental disorder.*

Exercise is essential for good quality sleep[112]*, especially if done in the morning or the afternoon. At night it can make it more difficult to fall asleep and should not be done. A sedentary lifestyle is bad for health. In fact, the World Health Organisation recommends a minimum of 3.5 hours of exercise a week. Most adults do not do this.*

Sleep environment: Besides these factors, there are others, such as sleeping in a room which is too hot or too cold, uncomfortable

---

[111] Baranwal N, Yu PK, Siegel NS. Sleep physiology, pathophysiology, and sleep hygiene. Prog Cardiovasc Dis. 2023 Mar-Apr;77:59-69. doi: 10.1016/j.pcad.2023.02.005. Epub 2023 Feb 24. PMID: 36841492.

[112] Firth J, Solmi M, Wootton RE, Vancampfort D, Schuch FB, Hoare E, Gilbody S, Torous J, Teasdale SB, Jackson SE, Smith L, Eaton M, Jacka FN, Veronese N, Marx W, Ashdown-Franks G, Siskind D, Sarris J, Rosenbaum S, Carvalho AF, Stubbs B. A meta-review of "lifestyle psychiatry": the role of exercise, smoking, diet and sleep in the prevention and treatment of mental disorders. World Psychiatry. 2020 Oct;19(3):360-380. doi: 10.1002/wps.20773. PMID: 32931092; PMCID: PMC7491615.

bed or pillows, noisy environments (air traffic, road traffic[113], machinery noise, noisy streets, noisy neighbours, discussions or fights at home, being in hospitalised or in intensive care units, etc), having light in the room because the blinds/curtains do not close, are equally inconvenient to sleep. White noise has however been proposed as a sleep aid to counter act the effects of noisy environments, but in a recent review the evidence upon sleep benefits was very low[114].

Sleep disturbers: Having to take care of somebody (baby, sick person), sleeping with pets, etc., may also be prejudicial.

Sleep stealers: TV, computers, play stations, mobile phones, messaging, social networks, etc. are, when used in excess and during the night, clear sleep stealers with negative sleep impacts. This has been proven for all ages: children/ adolescents[115] and adults[116]. Setting boundaries, utilizing parental controls, and demonstrating good screen behaviours are possible treatment strategies[117].

Sleep hygiene is a crucial part of life's daily hygiene.

[113] Smith MG, Cordoza M, Basner M. Environmental Noise and Effects on Sleep: An Update to the WHO Systematic Review and Meta-Analysis. Environ Health Perspect. 2022 Jul;130(7):76001. doi: 10.1289/EHP10197. Epub 2022 Jul 11. PMID: 35857401; PMCID: PMC9272916.

[114] Riedy SM, Smith MG, Rocha S, Basner M. Noise as a sleep aid: A systematic review. Sleep Med Rev. 2021 Feb;55:101385. doi: 10.1016/j.smrv.2020.101385. Epub 2020 Sep 9. PMID: 33007706.

[115] LeBourgeois MK, Hale L, Chang AM, Akacem LD, Montgomery-Downs HE, Buxton OM. Digital Media and Sleep in Childhood and Adolescence. Pediatrics. 2017 Nov;140(Suppl 2):S92-S96. doi: 10.1542/peds.2016-1758J. PMID: 29093040; PMCID: PMC5658795.

[116] Lakerveld J, Mackenbach JD, Horvath E, Rutters F, Compernolle S, Bárdos H, De Bourdeaudhuij I, Charreire H, Rutter H, Oppert JM, McKee M, Brug J. The relation between sleep duration and sedentary behaviours in European adults. Obes Rev. 2016 Jan;17 Suppl 1:62-7. doi: 10.1111/obr.12381. PMID: 26879114.

[117] Muppalla SK, Vuppalapati S, Reddy Pulliahgaru A, Sreenivasulu H. Effects of Excessive Screen Time on Child Development: An Updated Review and Strategies for Management. Cureus. 2023 Jun 18;15(6):e40608. doi: 10.7759/cureus.40608. PMID: 37476119; PMCID: PMC10353947.

9. SLEEP IS A WASTE OF TIME

Sleeping is a waste of time.

I love life. I can't stop. There is so much to do.

I am doing a Business Management course and working in accountancy.

With the degree I should be able to get a better job. I am also doing an AI course. You can't do anything nowadays without knowing about that.

I get up between 6:30 and 7:00 am, I am at work by 8:00 am. I have a coffee in the coffee shop and work straight through until 5:00 pm.

Lunch? I eat in a little greasy soup, standing at the counter to save time. Then, depending on the day, I go to language classes Mondays and Wednesdays from 6:00 to 7:00 pm, and Management classes Tuesdays and Thursdays from 6:00 to 10:00 pm and Mondays, Wednesdays and Fridays from 7:00 pm to 10:00 pm

Working out? I don't have time.

I have dinner between 10:00 and 11:00 pm and lie down for 1 or 2 hours because I must study.

At weekends I must study and on Saturdays I have a part-time job. I write stuff for a company.

Dating? I just don't have time for it. That will have to come later.

On Sundays I go and watch football and sometimes play with my friends.

Lately I have not been doing that so much, as most of them have got married and don't have leisure time anymore.

Dating before? I had relationships but they never went well. I am just going to think about that when I finish the Management course and have a more regular lifestyle. Now I must work and pay off the debts I have taken on.

Of course, I still live with my parents, but I have bought a house and a car, and I have to pay them off. The house is an investment and the car a necessity.

I can't stop. I get ill if I do nothing. I like my life and I like working.

In holidays I get nervous easily. I must be always doing something. It's just that now I get headaches. I get them upon wake up and they get worse by the end of the day. I feel very irritable.

And my memory is not as good as it used to be. Every now and then I cannot remember what I must do; in the past I was just like a machine. I did not need help. I knew everything to the last detail. Sometimes I want to sleep but I just can't do it. I don't want to sleep a lot; sleeping is a waste of time. I know you don't agree but that is what I think. But now I can't even sleep in those few hours...

This individual is a workaholic. He cannot live without working and does not like holidays. Taking him away from work brings on anxiety, distress and depression.

He has a chronic lack of sleep. Sleep deprivation in the early stages may bring on a certain pleasure: the person manages to do things that others cannot do and feels this to be stimulating: "I am better than the others".

Sleep deprivation can be tolerated for some years, but after a period, which varies from person to person, the first effects start to be noticed: memory problems, irritability, inability to sleep, headaches. From then on, the path towards becoming more serious is progressive and rapid.

His personal life takes second place. All your efforts and energy are concentrated on work and on professional and economic success. There is not even any effort to live independently on your own – you accept living with your parents.

The pleasures of life are highly reduced.

Workaholism is a serious problem[118]. A distinction must be made between excessive work (working too many hours) and workaholism (addiction to work). Addiction is a neuropsychological disorder characterized by a persistent and intense urge to use a drug or engage in a behaviour that produces natural reward, despite substantial harm and other negative consequences. Workaholism is a compulsive and extreme need to work, characterized by an unrelenting drive to work hours on end, take on more work responsibility and prioritize work over different areas of life, such as family and friends[119].

There are several scales to measure workaholism: The Work Addiction Risk Test, the Workaholism Battery, the Dutch Work Addiction Scale, the Bergen Work Addiction Scale

Workaholism_has mental and physical health consequences, namely: anxiety, depression, burnout, sleep problems, cardiovascular disease, lower life satisfaction, work-family conflicts, marital dissatisfaction, work related accidents, negative organizational outcomes and job dissatisfaction.

There is a lot in life besides work and voluntary sleep deprivation.

As time goes by you will pay for this work addiction dearly.

---

[118] Barbosa NS, Lira JAC, Ribeiro AAA, Rocha EPD, Galdino MJQ, Fernandes MA. Factors associated with workaholism in nurses' mental health: integrative review. Rev Lat Am Enfermagem. 2024 Jul 29;32:e4218. doi: 10.1590/1518-8345.7046.4218. PMID: 39082501; PMCID: PMC11295265.

[119] Andersen FB, Djugum MET, Sjåstad VS and Pallesen S (2023) The prevalence of workaholism: a systematic review and meta-analysis. Front. Psychol. 14:1252373. doi: 10.3389/fpsyg.2023.1252373

10. I DON'T HAVE TIME TO SLEEP

Husband - I have already said that I am not going to bed now. I still need to work a little bit more. Pleasant dreams and turn out the light. I don't have time to sleep.

I've got a meeting at 8 am tomorrow with Smith to prepare the reception for the overseas visitors. They are arriving at... actually, I can't remember. I am not sure if it is at 10 or at 11 am. Good grief, I used to have a wonderful memory but it's starting to fail me. The activity plan is done, but the strategy is still barely defined.

Puff... Eh!? What happened?

The computer crashed. I've lost everything... did I save it?

No... I didn't... What a drag!

Wife - Well, calm down and sort it out. What time is it?

Husband - It's 3:30 am and I have lost everything I did after the activity plan. I'm not going to manage to do it!

Wife - Do you want a glass of milk?

Husband - No, shut up! Leave me alone, I've got to finish this.

Wife - Please come and lie down, this is killing you! This is not life, this is nothing.

Husband - I told you I want to be left alone. Go and lie down. I'll finish this in a jiffy. I can still have 3 or 4 hours of sleep.

STARTEGIC PLEN — The objcetive is ......

Husband - What am I writing? This makes no sense. The ideas are not flowing. I am going to lie down. I have to sleep and remove this turmoil from my head. Maybe I can do better tomorrow.

Next morning...

Wife - Wake up! You asked me to wake you at 7am. What is your day going to be like? I've brought you breakfast.

Husband - Are you angry? I am sorry for shouting yesterday but I was really unlucky. I have got to go in early to do everything all over again. My head feels heavy. I don't feel like eating.

Wife - Do you want to take a pill? You can't leave without eating something!

Husband - Are you still angry?

Wife - Of course I am. I am angry and very worried. You're fat. You have daily headaches; you are forgetful and irritable, and it seems like you don't live here anymore. You get home late, never before 10 pm. Dinner is always waiting for you, cold. I can't handle having dinner so late and sleeping so little. I try and make up for it with an afternoon nap, but not you, it's just work, work, work! You are leaving work later and later!

Husband - Stop. I have a headache.

Wife - Of course you have a headache and worse it will become with your present stress. I heard on the TV that it causes heart attacks. You look like a zombie, and you do nothing but work, both during the week and at weekends. We haven't been on holiday for 3 years. When are you going to stop?

Husband - In the current circumstances I don't have any choice. Just a little more time and then everything will change.

..... Outside in the traffic... Sound of horns.

Wife - Phew, what a fright! You're crazy! You were going to hit that car! You look like death warmed up.

Husband - That guy does not know how to drive. He must have taken his licence on the examiners' day off.

Wife - Pete it was your fault. Calm down. At least you did not hit him. Calm down. You are acting crazily! Calm down please. Tomorrow I am booking an appointment with the doctor! This is not normal!

Husband - You know very well that I cannot stop. We have got the mortgage to pay, the loan on the car, the kids' school. I must hold a bit longer.

Wife - What you must do is calm down. If you get sick you won't earn anything.

Many people, whether male or female, have a tiring lifestyles and excessive workloads which are harmful to their health[120]. Many people's day-to-day life is just an accumulation of mistakes:

- ***The daily stress – traffic congestion, unstable employment or job at risk, the need to increase your professional worth, financial commitments, etc...***
- ***Sleep reduction – you sleep less than ever and go to bed late.***
- ***Bad food habits – leaving home without having breakfast, eating quickly during the day, having a late dinner which is sometimes the only meal of the day.***
- ***Excessive work and worries – Working too much throughout extended hours, with many deadlines, multitasking, successive interruptions, responsibilities and conflicts, not pausing during work, not having free time during weekends and holidays, etc.***

---

[120] Caldwell JA, Caldwell JL, Thompson LA, Lieberman HR. Fatigue and its management in the workplace. Neurosci Biobehav Rev. 2019 Jan;96:272-289. doi: 10.1016/j.neubiorev.2018.10.024. Epub 2018 Nov 2. PMID: 30391406.

The consequences are terrible, but since they appear insidiously, they are hardly noticed. When your body alerts you, sometimes it is too late.

The consequences are:

- *Insomnia, sleep deprivation and memory problems.*
- *Burnout, depression, anxiety, irritability, stress*
- *Obesity, diabetes, hypertension, cardiovascular and stroke risks.*
- *Fatigue, tiredness, lapses, errors and work-related accidents*
- *Reduced libido and sexual problems*

The first signs of sleep deprivation are irritability and memory or concentration problems.

Sleep deprivation carries also the risk of hypertension due to increased cortisol secretion (the stress hormone); there is a risk of diabetes due to increased insulin resistance.

You get fat because sleep deprivation reduces the production of leptin (which reduces appetite) and increases the production of orexin and ghrelin (which stimulate the appetite). Having a late dinner coincides with the production of "ghrelin" by the stomach which facilitates food absorption. Stress, in turn, increases the production of endogenous cortisol, which can also lead to obesity, mainly the so-called "buffalo type" obesity, with greater adiposity in the neck, abdomen and thorax.

Everything together leads to an increase in weight, which, in turn, brings with it cardiovascular risks.

Burnout is a state of exhaustion, fatigue, and frustration due to a professional activity that fails to produce the expected expectations. It causes damage at a cognitive, emotional, and attitudinal level, which translates into negative behaviour towards work, peers, users, and the professional role itself[121]

With time the patient, depressed and exhausted, is no longer able to work; this incapacity is often prolonged, and 100% recovery is not always possible.

Just like high-performance athletes, those who must work hard, must be extra careful with their food habits, lifestyle and sleep patterns.

Your body is your working tool. If you ruin it, you can't work.

[121] Edú-Valsania S, Laguía A, Moriano JA. Burnout: A Review of Theory and Measurement. Int J Environ Res Public Health. 2022 Feb 4;19(3):1780. doi: 10.3390/ijerph19031780. PMID: 35162802; PMCID: PMC8834764.

11. I CAN'T BE QUIET. I MUST DO SEVERAL THINGS AT THE SAME TIME

I cannot stop. At work I interrupt everybody with questions and work control. "Did you phone client X?", "Did you deliver item Y?". Idem with my kids, I do not allow they are doing nothing.

My wife says I am connected to electricity.

I must be always doing something. Doing nothing is not for me. I almost panic.

During work I do many things at the same, nowadays this is a must, and in the evening, I do several things simultaneously: the PC, the TV, some music. I must have all "channels" busy otherwise I don't sleep, because I will be worried with what I have not done.

I don't sleep well. I have no problems falling asleep, but I wake up at 3 or 4 am, and after that, either I don't sleep or start a sleep/awakening state which I don't know whether I am awake or asleep.

Recently, I felt tired, I would say, exhausted. I forgot two essential appointments, and shout with one co-worker, and put the car keys in the fridge. I recognise I need help.

We're in the age of multitasking. The aim is to do a lot of different things at the same time, the more the better. This fashion took!

The housewives have been doing it for a while, with one child on the lap while scolding the other, and cooking lunch as well as thinking of a groceries list.

Housekeepers dusting off with one hand, while answering the mobile phone with the other, do it.

The intellectuals with their PC, TV, MP3 and cell phones, while attempting to erase any free space for any reverie, do it.

Children switching from toy to toy, not to get bored, do it.

Teenagers with their iPad, SMS, play station while they study for the following day's test, do it.

Those who believe in the benefits of physical exercise, walk miles or kilometres on the treadmill or on the elliptical machine while watching TV, speaking on the cell phone, reading reports or studying professional matters, do it.

The executives with multiple cell phones: the company's, the home phone, the one for the special clients, plus their iPads, and the notes passed along to their secretaries, do it.

The politicians, with multiple phones, their PC and many counsellors and secretaries, preparing strategic questions, giving news concerning "pressing" affairs, or preparing schedules for tomorrow's meetings, do it.

Journalists, salesmen, businessmen, doctors, lawyers, veterinarians, pharmaceuticals, policemen...almost everyone does it.

So many people are buzzing around in this cacophony of tasks, running like tired horses, without knowing or wondering about the purpose of the race.

Multitasking demands and work interruptions are the new stressors.

The Autonomous Nervous System has two components with somewhat opposite actions: the Sympathetic and the Parasympathetic; the former is a biological marker of stress responses together with the hypothalamic-pituitary-adrenal axis and the immune system. Increase in Sympathetic activity is a risk for high blood pressure, which can lead to cardiovascular or renal disease; to hyperglycaemia which can lead to type II diabetes, anxiety and depression, and obesity, metabolic syndrome, and bowel disease.

Sympathetic Nervous System reactivity (measured objectively by salivary alpha-amylase) changes significantly in work interruptions, parallel dual-tasking, and multitasking conditions; there were no changes in the hypothalamic-pituitary adrenal axis and short-term immune response[122].

Multitasking and work interruptions affect the brain

I usually say that these systematic oscillations between tasks are like walking in a zigzag, with successive refocusing periods, for every single task, which leads to more effort and inevitable fatigue. Zigzagging takes longer than going in a straight line. Furthermore, one does not think straight, nor does one ponder on each subject.

Task switching increases error rates!

In functional terms our brain has no possibility to activate the "default mode network", essential to adequate brain functioning. The consequences are lapses, errors, attention deficits, memory problems and ultimately sleep dysfunction.

The issue at hand is that, after a systematic bombardment of the brain and senses, people want to have a good night's sleep because they are tired. Impossible!

Don't fool yourselves; the brain is like a muscle: when fatigue is excessive, it cannot rest and...farewell Sleep!

Sleep comes with tranquility, silence and comfort.

---

[122] Becker L, Kaltenegger HC, Nowak D, Weigl M, Rohleder N. Biological stress responses to multitasking and work interruptions: A randomized controlled trial. Psychoneuroendocrinology. 2023 Oct;156:106358. doi:10.1016/j.psyneuen.2023.106358. Epub 2023 Aug 2. PMID: 37542740.

Little Advices:

First, it's important for you to accept that you are multitasking.

Then, realize which tasks you must really do and schedule breaks.

However...

Should you feel a lot of adrenaline because you are able to multitask so much, you should know that adrenaline in excess damages your heart, memory and reasoning.

If you're one of those persons that need to be "online" all the time, find several periods of time during your day that you are "offline". Surely the world does not rest on your shoulders all the time...

If you work in an open space, and are continuously being interrupted, try to find a way for that not to happen...at least during two continuous periods of the day.

If you are in a leadership position, and are always being interrupted by your co-workers, stipulate rules to be interrupted only during selected periods of your day.

If we are constantly interrupted by your clients stipulate attending hours.

If you are in a leadership position or must do intellectual work schedule your day in slots so that you do one thing at a time and are NOT interrupted during demanding tasks requiring focused attention.

Don't spend your whole day plugged to your cell phone, and don't send text messages or e-mails during your scheduled breaks.

Skip the announcements of "new mail" "new message" in the phone and email

If you don't know how, learn to spend several moments of your day in pause, doing nothing. You will progressively become calmer and more imaginative.

Whichever the situation in your daily routine that calls for multitasking, learn how to protect yourself from it.

Take small brakes

Meditation techniques, so popular nowadays, are meant to quiet our minds and focus our thoughts, in an opposite perspective to multitasking.

Would Da Vinci or Einstein have amounted to anything if they spent the entire day plugged to their cell phones or answering coworkers?

Are you an octopus with eight arms?

In the Bible the Creation is described in succession, one day after the other, and even God rested at the 7th day.

E. Risks of Bad or Unregulated Sleep

1. RISKS FOR YOUR HEART

SEVERAL TIME ZONES IN THE SAME DAY

James - These relaxing moments are quite unusual. I always feel a bit anxious during holidays. I miss the working place adrenaline

Jules - Me too; the bird songs do not replace the working brou-ah-ah and its endless needs.

Jim - Are you definitively crazy or just dependent?

Jules – I am not crazy, but I am certainly dependent of my work. My doctor told me that and asked me whether I would like to have an infarct at an airport, somewhere in the world …

Jim – Why did he tell you that? Dying at an airport is certainly not fun

Jules – Well I travel a lot, and mostly among different time zones which change constantly. To explain better: I live in the Philippines, one of my businesses is in Shanghai, another in India and another office in South Africa. I wake up in …, ie, Philippines, I travel to Shanghai for the afternoon and sleep somewhere in India; the next day I might go to South Africa and return home.

James – Well, without travelling in fact I also travel. At 3am I start the negotiations in the Shangai stocks, at 8am I connect to the Berlin stocks and during the afternoon I am between Berlin and New York. The important is also the closure time at about 1 am, here and soon after open the Asian markets. So you see I have all the time zones in my head, even without travelling

Jim – You would rather die at any of your locations between so many time zones? Which is your limit?

James – There are no limits, dear friend. Do you remember our old times. Jules and I willing to conquer the world and become rich ...

Jules – Ten per cent more every year ...

James- We managed, didn't we? I have my Rolls, my yacht and my Monet and Jules is flooded with money

Jules – You are also flooded with wives. How many so far? 5 or 6?

James – Only five! After the fifth divorce I start realizing it was too expensive and changed the paradigm. Just girlfriends, with gorgeous bodies, and anxious for sex and fun

Jules – Associated with some sniffing materials, I imagine ...

James – Humm ...sometimes. Hey Jim, did you get what you wanted from life?

Jules – What did you really wanted; we never understand you.

Jim was silent. His life was not glamourous; he was not rich and was working every day to get a medium low salary. He had only one wife and three kids. He loved her and enjoyed having sex with her after all these years. He was proud of his children and enjoys being with them and discussing with them several aspects of daily life. He had a small garden with the most beautify camellias, while Mary was planting kitchen herbs. They had a cat and a turtle, interacting strangely at the garden. He was sure his friends would find him a "silly and uninteresting person" with the strange and unprofitable attitude of rescuing wild animals and treating them in a farm somewhere. So he kept all that for himself and answer in a loud voice.

Jim – I have a normal life with my family

James — Good so, congratulations! We will meet again in 10 years, do you both agree

Ten years latter

James looked a bit strange; the implanted hair was not enough to hide he was becoming bold, and the face was strange, as if some unusual and unlikely muscle contractions were appearing under his skin, with no correlation with any facial expression.

Jules looked much older full of wrinkles and grey hair, and moving a bit slow as if his limbs were weak; he look sad with a dark shadow over his eyes.

James was unrestful, unable to be quiet, looking around as something was persecuting him

Jim — Any problem with you?

James — No, you know, I had a stupid relation with some splendorous blond, who had the silly idea of denouncing stock activities. You know people doesn't like to lost money in the stock market: They only like to win. The tax department is after me some unsatisfied clients also. I have to take care, that's it.

Jim — And your Rolls and your Monet?

James — Well things got complicated; I had to stop. It was strange, during one week I win a lot, as if some little intuition was leading me to the valuable markets, but the week after, fully confident with the previous success, I took some wrong decisions.

Jules — Some people say that your wrong decisions started during the successful week, which was not so successful after all.

James — Gossip; people is inventing things

Jim remembered some news in the newspapers and understood they referred to his friend.

Jim – And you; Jules, how is life going?

Jules – I had a heart attack at the airport, and nowadays I am flooded, not with money but with medication. Heart, Cholesterol, Diabetes, Uric acid, Stomach everything goes wrong, together with my knees, which prevent any speed in my legs. An old man, not disguised as he is.

James – I am also taking medication, somewhat equal to years plus the shrink medication. Drugs to be calm, not to depress, to stand the stress, to counteract drugs and alcohol. I am a pharmacy; a walking pharmacy. And you Jim? How are things going?

Jim – I am OK, with my normal life, my family, healthy, no medication...

This small story deals with three different aspects, which either simultaneously or independently converge to sleep quality

One is CHRONOBIOLOGY – jetlag symptoms only arose in human history when there were jets making possible to travel several time zones in a short time; just remember Jules Verne[123] novel published in 1873 and the Best picture Award academy film in 1956: "Around the World in 80 days[124]"

When we travel several times zones in a short time a desynchrony occurs between our internal clock and the clock of the present time zone. This phenomenon is called jetlag. The impact is different whether we travel east (stronger negative impact) or west (milder

---

[123] Jules Verne is a French novelist and poet (1828-1905)
[124] Around the World in 80 days- There are several movies with this name
- German silent movie , directed and produced by Richard Oswald and starring Conrad Veidt, Anita Berber, and Reinhold Schünzel in 1919
- American movie, Directors - Michael Anderson and John Farrow; Stars: David Niven, Cantinflas, Shirley MacLaine in 1956
- American movie, remake from 1956 movie; Director – Frank Coraci; Stars: Jackie Chan, Steve Coogan, Cécile de France and Jim Broadbent in 2004
- French animated comedy movie in 2021 directed by Samuel Tourneux

negative impact) and depends on the number of crossed time zones (the more the worse).

This is the case of Jules

There is another type of jetlag, called social jetlag, which occurs in most societies and individuals according to alternating schedules in workdays and free days. So, people might have jetlag without travelling. Taken to an extreme Jack circadian clock must change to external time, without travelling, adapting to the stock markets in different time zones across the world. The same occurs in businesspeople with clients in several continents.

Jetlag symptoms are nausea, irritability, anxiety, changed bowel habits (constipation or diarrhoea), difficulty concentrating, lower alertness, sleepiness, not feeling very well, headaches, feeling low.

The risks of chronic circadian misalignment are: diminished attention, memory, and executive function, psychosocial disruption, impaired emotional regulation, increased risk of depression, obesity, diabetes, heart disease, auto-immune disorders, metabolic syndrome, stroke, sepsis, intestinal inflammation, cancers and early death.

The other is EXCESSIVE WORK – which is associated with increased risk of high blood pressure, heart and cardiovascular diseases, burnout, depression, anxiety, insomnia.

The third one is HAPPINESS AND WELL BEING – The idea of and Jack implies happiness centred in wealth and success

However, studies have shown that : (a) people in richer nations are happier than people in poorer nations; (b) increases in national wealth within developed nations have not, over recent decades, been associated with increases in SWB; (c) within-nation differences in wealth show only small positive correlations with happiness; (d)increases in personal wealth do not typically result in increased happiness; and (e) people who strongly desire wealth and money are more unhappy than those who do not (f) financial status was more correlated with life satisfaction in poorer nations than wealthier nations[125].

People who have strong social relationships tend to report higher levels of well-being; subjective reports of relationship quality and relationship satisfaction tend to exhibit the highest correlations with subjective well-being. Marital status is one of the strongest demographic predictors of happiness. Married people consistently report higher levels of happiness than single people, who report greater happiness than the widowed, divorced, or separated.

Just stop and think a little bit! Is it worth?

[125] Ryan RM, Deci EL. On happiness and human potentials: a review of research on hedonic and eudaimonic well-being. Annu Rev Psychol. 2001;52:141-66. doi:10.1146/annurev.psych.52.1.141. PMID: 11148302.

2. ACCIDENT RISKS

WHEN I WOKE UP, I WAS UNDER A LORRY

I had an accident because I fell asleep.

I didn't realize anything. I was on the motorway, on a straight road.

It seems that I hit the central barrier and then I went offline and ploughed into the back of a TIR lorry.

Despite everything I did not notice anything.

I woke up with the feeling that the roof of my bedroom had fallen on my head. It was the roof of the car which was crushed during the accident.

Happily, I only had a little scratch on my hand, and I did not kill anybody.

It is a bit too late to ask for medical advice

Falling asleep at the wheel is very dangerous. Somnolence at the wheel is more dangerous than alcohol. There are various situations that can cause this:

1. *People who have excessive sleepiness because they have a sleep disorder, such as sleep apnoea[126] or narcolepsy.*
2. *People who have excessive sleepiness because they are chronically sleep deprived. Sleeping less than 5 hours increases the risk of accidents, and with less than 3 hours the risk is even greater[127].*

---

[126] Karimi M, Hedner J, Lombardi C, Mcnicholas WT, Penzel T, Riha RL, Rodenstein D, Grote L; Esada Study Group. Driving habits and risk factors for traffic accidents among sleep apnea patients--a European multi-centre cohort study. JSleep Res. 2014 Dec;23(6):689-699. doi: 10.1111/jsr.12171. Epub 2014 Jul 7. PMID: 25040185.

[127] Basit H, Damhoff TC, Huecker MR. Sleeplessness and Circadian Disorder. 2023 Jun 13. In: StatPearls [Internet]. Treasure Island (FL): StatPearls Publishing; 2024 Jan–. PMID: 30480971.

3. *People with poor sleep[128]*

4. *People who drive at daybreak. At 4:00 am the risk of an accident increases 80%.*

5. *People who have excessive sleepiness because they are taking drugs, psychoactive or hypnotic medication[129].*

6. *Alcohol and sleep deprivation/excessive sleepiness cause additional effects, substantially increasing the risk of accidents.*

7. *The high point for accidents by young adults is, for these reasons, greater in the early mornings of Fridays and Saturdays.*

8. *People, who often dose or nap when driving, have an increased risk of having fatal accidents both for themselves and for others.*

9. *Night shift workers have an added risk of accidents when returning home at the end of their night shift.*

10. *Accidents often occur near home, when almost there, because you have been holding off the sleepiness... "nearly there" ... until it becomes irresistible and unavoidable.*

11. *In the early morning, accidents are not caused by falling asleep but rather caused by fatigue, which is related to lack of sleep, and the consequent lack of wakefulness and delays in one's reflexes.*

Sleepy drivers use various strategies to keep driving: opening the window, playing music loudly, hitting their face, taking off their

---

[128] Philip P, Chaufton C, Orriols L, Lagarde E, Amoros E, Laumon B, Akerstedt T, Taillard J, Sagaspe P. Complaints of Poor Sleep and Risk of Traffic Accidents: A Population-Based Case-Control Study. PLoS One. 2014 Dec 10;9(12):e114102. doi: 10.1371/journal.pone.0114102. PMID: 25494198; PMCID: PMC4262408.

[129] Abdoli N, Sadeghi Bahmani D, Farnia V, Alikhani M, Golshani S, Holsboer-Trachsler E, Brand S. Among substance-abusing traffic offenders, poor sleep and poor general health predict lower driving skills but not slower reaction times. Psychol Res Behav Manag. 2018 Nov 9;11:557-566. doi: 10.2147/PRBM.S173946. PMID: 30519130; PMCID: PMC6233697.

shoes. However, there are no effective strategies, since excessive sleepiness is irresistible.

The first signs are an increase in blinking, weaving and driving off the road.

When the sleepiness is not so great, caffeine can help. When it is great, it is better to stop and to sleep a little and only go back driving when you feel you have recovered, or not drive at all.

Excessive sleepiness is the first cause of fatal accidents. Accidents due to excessive sleepiness have the following characteristics:

- *They occur in inexplicable situations (straight roads, good visibility, etc.).*
- *They happen most often in the early morning.*
- *The driver does not carry out any manoeuvres to avoid the accident.*
- *There are no other plausible explanations for the accident. News stories concerning accidents of this kind are unfortunately frequent. It is vital to change these negative accident statistics.*

If you are sleepy, do not drive. Sleepiness at the wheel can kill.

3. OVERWEIGHT RISKS

WHEN I WAKE UP IN THE MORNING THERE ARE CRUMBS IN THE ROOM

My husband told me to come to your clinic.

At night I get up without really noticing, go to the kitchen and eat whatever is in the fridge. I eat biscuits, bread, fruit or whatever. I have eaten dog food which was being kept in the fridge. You can't imagine how much fun they made of me!

In the morning, I know something happened because I see that look on my husband's face and hear the giggles of my daughter.

They joke with me, and say it is impossible I don't realise what is happening! But I really don't... I have at the most, a vague idea that something has happened.

"Are you fatter?"

"Yes, I do regular diets, and I am the fatter/thinner type, overall I got 11lbs extra. Sometimes I get the food munchies, even when awake, and eat everything in front of me: everything that is bad for you: chocolates, cakes, sausages, *chorizo*, cheese, and things with many calories."

This is sleep-related eating disorder[130]. *Patients tend to eat foods full of calories, or sometimes even incredible things: leftovers, animal food, etc., but they do not remember doing this.*

What is important is to solve any situations involving stress and investigate if there is a specific food disorder, such as bulimia or

---

[130] Lipford MC, Auger RR. Sleep-Related Eating Disorder. Sleep Med Clin. 2024 Mar;19(1):55-61. doi: 10.1016/j.jsmc.2023.10.013. Epub 2023 Nov 29. PMID: 38368069.

anorexia, which is common both in the patients and members of their families.

The treatment is then contextualised within the treatment for this eating disorder.

This can also, as with the previous case, be linked to Periodic Limb Movements, depression or stressful situations. There is often a family history of eating disorders (anorexia, bulimia, etc.).

The increased weight risk due to sleep problems can have several mechanisms:

- Ingestion of the caloric foods at night, since during the night food absorption is higher.
- Being awaken at night (working, playing games, screens at night) and eating several snacks. The mechanism is dual: awake at night increases orexin and ghrelin levels while reducing leptin production, which together with the caloric food simply put on pounds
- Short and long sleep are both associated with increasing weight risk
- Excessive Stress and excessive work, are usually associated to sleep curtailment, while stress increases endogenous cortisol production; the final consequence is increased weight

If your weight is increasing pay attention to your sleep

If want to loose weight don't forget to sleep well

4. CHRONIC DISEASE RISKS

EVERYTHING HURTS, EVERYTHING IS TIRING

I don't have the strength for anything. Everything hurts. It's either my back, or my elbow, or my wrists, or my knees.

Mark doesn't believe me when I complain and does not pay any attention!

Neither do the doctors. "The examinations are normal".

Pills help a bit but who says I can sleep at night? Moving around in the bed is a torment.

The other day I lowered myself and had to stay squatting, without being able to get up again. They had to help me. It's martyrdom!

I don't have the strength for anything. I don't know if it's the pains or what it is, but how can I live my life? I walk a few steps and I'm exhausted. I haven't got the strength for anything. Tidying and cooking are such a torment. I do everything bit by bit. I wash the dishes and sit down, I stack the pots and stop, I hoover the floor and start sweating.

I don't know what I am going to do with my life!

I look at the mess in the living room and I feel like crying. I would love to see everything tidied, clean, shining...

What is certain is that I really feel like crying, of closing myself within a hole and waiting for all this to go way, to get my strength back and the pains to just disappear. If at least I could know what it is I've got!

It's been like this for 3 years.

I used to be able to handle everything. Then there were the repairs on the house, the death of my mother, the death of my father-in-law, the mess of the inheritance, the changes, working until so late, and I with my happy face putting up with everything. Mark knew that he could count on me.

They were crazy years of worry and work and then it seemed that something snapped, something broke and I have been in this state ever since.

I thought I was tired, but it was just the same or even worse after the holidays.

The dust from the kitchen dries my eyes and my mouth feels like sandpaper.

If I could at least sleep. Nights are such a sacrifice; tossing and turning, my head can't stop, trying and trying to sleep in vain. Sometimes I hardly know if I am awake, sleeping or if I have been dreaming.

I'm going to eat something. I must be careful about what I eat.

Now everything does harm and every now and then I get diarrhoea.

I am so tired! I just can't do anything. Climbing the stairs is so tiring, walking is so tiring, having a bath is so tiring, washing my head is so tiring. I feel like crap.

I feel so cold! It is such a lovely day, and I feel so cold.

I have Mark's clothes to iron. Two shirts. I can't complain. Better just to clench my teeth and get everything done. I'll manage, I must. If he gets back and dinner is still to be cooked I will hear some more "home truths". "There goes the invalid convalescing": of course I'm an invalid. Everything hurts. My head feels heavy, I don't have the strength to even raise a feather, I can't sleep, and I just feel like crawling into a hole, disappearing and bursting out crying.

If he gets at me, I will really shout, I'll make a scene; he won't be able to turn away from.

He just does not respect what I am suffering, not him or anyone.

My mother says I am crazy. He is the one who tells her and complains. He twists everything, like in the argument yesterday:

"You've been on sick leave for 1 month, we have spent a fortune on pills and exams. I've paid for I don't know how many medical appointments and you're always the same. You're not even good for anything in bed. - "I'm tired", "I've got a headache", "I just don't feel like it". Just get yourself fixed because I can't take much more of this".

It was an argument and a half. What is certain is that I just don't feel like doing anything. What if he finds somebody else?

Oh God, what would I do? It's hopeless!

Complaining of aches and pains all over the body, fatigue, insomnia and depression suggest the possibility of fibromyalgia[131]. Fibromyalgia often arises following persistent bouts of stress but there are also familiar tendencies.

Fibromyalgia is a multifactorial disorder, the cause of which is still unknown and symptoms for which include the following:

- *Bilateral diffuse musculoskeletal pains, above and below the waist.*
- *The presence of pain in at least 11 of 18 designated tender points.*
- *Chronic fatigue from daily tasks.*
- *Insomnia, with difficulty in sleeping and a sleeping-whilst-awake sensation.*
- *Restless legs syndrome*
- *Depression, anxiety and irritability.*
- *Headaches.*
- *Memory lapses and "brain fog"*

131 Bair MJ, Krebs EE. Fibromyalgia. Ann Intern Med. 2020 Mar 3;172(5):ITC33-ITC48. doi: 10.7326/AITC202003030. PMID: 32120395.

- *Dry mouth and mucous membranes.*
- *Bowel disturbances and irritable bowel syndrome.*
- *Sexual dysfunction*
- *Difficulties in controlling temperature, chiefly in cold environments.*
- *Symptom fluctuations throughout the day in line with one's circadian rhythm.*
- *Possibility of being linked to other rheumatic and medical illnesses.*

Despite being commonly considered as a psychological disease, there are characteristic and very common organic disturbances in fibromyalgia, namely:

- *Alterations in sleep, in terms of alpha delta sleep and the frequent presence of restless legs or periodic movements, and sleep apnea or upper airway resistance syndrome*
- *Disturbances in the pituitary gland and hypothalamus stem.*
- *Disturbances in the central processing of pain.*
- *Alterations in the metabolism of lipids with high cholesterol.*

One of the problems of fibromyalgia is its low recognition on the part of health professionals and the community, with there still being doctors who state that it is something that does not exist, and has arisen from peoples' imagination or is just a psychiatric disorder.

Fibromyalgia is, however, a well-defined disease with its own diagnostic criteria established by the American College of Rheumatology in 1990.

Treatment for fibromyalgia is multifactorial.

It is important to change your way of dealing with things and with life, recognising your limitations so as to be able to do what you can and thus avoid exhaustion. Just as those going out to sea in a motorboat have to take enough petrol for the outward and inward journey, patients with fibromyalgia should calculate what they can do without exhausting their abilities.

It is important to avoid unnecessary efforts, such as walking with excessive weight, doing tasks which are too heavy, etc.

The ability to carry out tasks varies throughout the day, and there are good moments and bad moments. It is important to take advantage of the good periods and stop during the bad periods.

Sleep should also be treated with medication and behavioural therapies adjusted to the disturbances encountered in each patient.

Fatigue can greatly improve with adjusted exercise programmes, which should also be tailored to each patient. Exercises and efforts which are too violent should be avoided, but exercise must be carried out.

It is important to drink plenty of water, something which many patients forget and the dryness of their eyes, if it is bothering them, can be solved with artificial tears.

Depression and irritability must be treated with pharmacological or psychotherapeutic support. Some patients have serious depressions which should be treated psychiatrically. Above all it is important to have an optimistic attitude. To say that a glass is half full is better than guaranteeing that it is half empty.

Food habits are also very important to avoid bad digestion, colic, and diarrhoeas.

It is equally important to treat the pain with specific medication which can be taken at night to improve night sleep and during the day to improve the quality of life.

There are currently new and promising drugs for the treatment of fibromyalgia. These drugs seek to simultaneously treat all the various main components of fibromyalgia: pain, fatigue, insomnia and depression, but, for the time being, none of the available options is effective for all of these elements and combinations are necessary.

Don't despair. It is possible to find solutions and support.

5. CANCER RISKS

I AM PAYING FOR WHAT I HAVE DONE

I was always working, no holidays, no family, WORK, WORK, WORK. Eating whenever possible, sleeping not much and whenever convenient, until one day I had to stop.

I enjoyed power, I enjoyed fame. I enjoyed earning money, but I used money to reinforce the firm and earn more money and more power.

Power and fame became the sweet perfume of my work. I was pleased, but perhaps not happy...

Whiskies to relax and smoking to think better.

People did not love me; they obeyed and collaborate.

I have no friends, but many people envy me and my life

From my own point of view, I went beyond my own dreams

I was pleased, but not happy

Everything was going smoothly until I had to stop with these 2 words: pancreatic cancer

From them a long way of boring things, NRMs, blood testing, PET scans

Two other words added: ductal adenocarcinoma

Pain increased and symptoms started, yellow, losing weight and weak

With surgery work become difficult, I was easily tired and with a terrible mood

I am too young to be tired.

In a recent dream I meet an old man, who was trying to tell me something, but vanished in the dream.

Maybe he wanted to tell me that I am going to die.

Pancreatic cancer is the fourth leading cause of cancer deaths in the United States [132]

This patient slept when convenient (circadian misalignment and sleep deprivation); to this he added other risk factors: tobacco, alcohol, poor nutrition, stress and excessive work.

Sleep deprivation impacts heavily upon the entire neuroendocrine-immune system complex that regulates cell proliferation, immune defense (including cytokine production and associated proinflammatory pathways), energy metabolism, bio logical response and adaptation to everyday stresses, and cognitive and physical performance [133].

Sleep deprivation leads to increase in inflammatory markers. Chronic low-level inflammatory states contribute to the development of many chronic medical conditions, including cardiovascular disease obesity, and cancer [133].

Oxidative stress appears to be an important factor in various human diseases. Oxidative stress occurs in a cell or tissue when the concentration of reactive oxygen species (ROS) generated exceeds the antioxidant capability of that cell. ROS is implicated

---

[132] Puckett Y, Garfield K. Pancreatic Cancer. [Updated 2022 Sep 26]. In: StatPearls [Internet]. Treasure Island (FL): StatPearls Publishing; 2024 Jan-. Available from: https://www.ncbi.nlm.nih.gov/books/NBK518996/

[133] Haus EL, Smolensky MH. Shift work and cancer risk: potential mechanistic roles of circadian disruption, light at night, and sleep deprivation. Sleep Med Rev. 2013 Aug;17(4):273-84. doi: 10.1016/j.smrv.2012.08.003. Epub 2012 Nov 6. PMID: 23137527.

in various phases of the carcinogenesis process and increases in states of sleep loss[134].

Power, Fame, Work, Money .... At the end of life do you take them with you?

---

[134]   Noguti J, Andersen ML, Cirelli C, Ribeiro DA. Oxidative stress, cancer, and sleep deprivation: is there a logical link in this association? Sleep Breath. 2013 Sep;17(3):905-10. doi: 10.1007/s11325-012-0797-9. Epub 2013 Feb 1. PMID: 23371889.

6. DEMENTIA RISKS

SHE WAS A SHORT SLEEPER

My mother was fantastic.

Very bright, people would say she was very intelligent.

Quite assertive, for her everything was either back or white, no grey zones.

Quite powerful, she would get what she wanted.

Quite careful with her appearance, the hair well done, well treated nails, cared hands.

Nice and elegant dresses.

She practiced gym, at home, upon awakening.

She worked a lot, until late at night, 1 or 2 am, but waking up quite early. At 6 am she was up.

Her coworkers could not stand her. They were exhausted and sleepy.

But she went on, working and solving problems, without a break

She was fantastic

But, one day, after her retirement, she lost herself in our neighbourhood. She phoned me asking for help, but she was quite close to home.

I think it was the first sign.

Then it was these strange lapses in memory: "Don't you remember? We were just talking about it half an hour ago."

She remembered well the past and could tell jokes about her position in Office. As she was intelligent, she could in the beginning use different paths to solve her drawbacks

But the "thing" was there! Memory lapses become more frequent, she became careless concerning her appearance and having critical attention lapses, burning her cooking, not closing a tap, etc.

It was then that we went to the doctor and the diagnosis was devastating.

According to the CDC[135] dementia involves "dysfunction in memory, attention, communication, reasoning judgment, problem solving and visual perception beyond typical age-related changes. In USA of those with at least 65 years of age, there is an estimated 5.0 million adults with dementia in 2014 and projected to be nearly 14 million by 2060". The worldwide increase in population age increases dementia prevalence.

There are several subtypes: Alzheimer's disease (AD), Vascular dementia, Lewy body dementia, Fronto-temporal dementia, Mixed dementia and Reversible causes[135].

In all types of dementia there are dysfunctional sleep-wake behaviours due pathogenic processes in the brain stem and the hypothalamus[136].

Sleep disturbances are common (60 to 70% of the people with cognitive impairment) and linked with poorer prognosis[137].

---

[135] What Is Dementia? | CDC

[136] Balan I, Bilger N, Saparov D, Hryb I, Abdyraimov A. Sleep Deprivation in Middle Age May Increase Dementia Risk: A Review. Cureus. 2023 Apr 11;15(4):e37425. doi: 10.7759/cureus.37425. PMID: 37181993; PMCID: PMC10174673.

[137] Wennberg AMV, Wu MN, Rosenberg PB, Spira AP. Sleep Disturbance, Cognitive Decline, and Dementia: A Review. Semin Neurol. 2017 Aug;37(4):395-406. doi: 10.1055/s-0037-1604351. Epub 2017 Aug 24. PMID: 28837986; PMCID: PMC5910033.

Sleep wake cycles are disrupted, either because along the 24h patients may be awake or asleep, by alternating periods, or because patients have an inverted sleep wake cycle and start sleeping during the day and are awake at night; another classical manifestation is <u>sundowning</u>, with confusion, agitation or disruptive behaviours occurring in the evening or night). These symptoms represent circadian disturbance likely associated with SCN (suprachiasmatic nucleus) degeneration.

Obstructive sleep apnoea is very common in dementia and contributes to poorer prognosis[137].

REM Sleep Disorder is common in Lewy body dementia.

Sleep deprivation is a modifiable risk factor of dementia. Self-report of shorter sleep duration (≤ 5 hours) is associated with 2.4 times the odds of AD, and self-reported longer sleep duration (≥ 9 hours) is associated with 2.8 times the odds of AD[137, 138].

Insomnia symptoms and sleep fragmentation are also associated with increased risk of mild cognitive impairment and dementia[137].

<u>Sleep well to prevent cognitive impairment</u>

---

[138]   Benito-León J, Bermejo-Pareja F, Vega S, Louis ED. Total daily sleep duration and the risk of dementia: a prospective population-based study. *Eur J Neurol.* 2009;16(09):990–997.

7. Lower Performance

I FAILED THE RACE COMPETITION

I was competing in a very important race.

My rank was quite high, so it was expected that I would win a podium classification

The pressure was high.

We arrived 2 days before, but the time difference between home and the competition city was 5 hours earlier, we travelled eastward.

I did not sleep well the first two days, the bed was OK, but the pillow was too high and too soft. I was a bit seasick, the stomach burning and some colic's.

I was tired, in a bad mood but start training.

A small, insignificant lesion in the left arm, which went away with massage

Training was painful. It was if I was training at night at home

The competition day I felt a bit better, but not 100% OK

The race started and at the end I was not among the 10 best athletes,

This result was devastating

Sleep is essential for all athletes, from all athletic specialities, since they are high performance individuals.

Poor sleep, sleep deprivation and circadian misalignment may deteriorate performance, while increasing the risk of lesions and accidents.

Poor sleep, stress, training and responsibilities will provoke fatigue and mental problems, while "opening the door" to burnout

Excessive training may induce athletes' burnout

Athletes are often forced to adhere to strict competition and travel schedules, while maintaining rigorous training; the travel schedules may induce circadian misalignment and, consequently, interfere with sleep[139].

Athletes often misinterpret insomnia symptoms as competition stress, and daytime sleepiness as fatigue[139]: both are, however, if persisting for 3 weeks and occurring more than 2 or 3 times per week, sleep disturbance symptoms

Recommendations[139] are:

Sleep hygiene

> *Regular sleep schedules for wake up and sleep,*
> *Consistent evening routine before bed*
> *Extend your sleep in case you are tired, or before a night of sleep deprivation*
> *Sleep adequately prior to competition*
> *Identify sleep disturbances and ask specialist advice*
> *Avoiding stimulants and distractions*
> *Getting natural light*
> *Avoiding blue light from computer and phone screens, since it disrupts melatonin release*
> *For evening competitions use blue blocker glasses when competition is over, and you go home/hotel*
> *Stress reduction and meditation*
> *Proper nutrition*

[139] Vitale KC, Owens R, Hopkins SR, Malhotra A. Sleep Hygiene for Optimizing Recovery in Athletes: Review and Recommendations. Int J Sports Med. 2019 Aug;40(8):535-543. doi: 10.1055/a-0905-3103. Epub 2019 Jul 9. PMID: 31288293; PMCID: PMC6988893.

Training

Avoid excessive training
Avoid evening training since it may induce sleep onset delay and phase shifts your sleep
Take pauses

Travel (see: I am flying East, to Lisbon)

In case of travel consider the associated jetlag and get personalized advice
Consider the time of lower incapacity as a function of time zones travelled
Consider the jetlag symptoms
Use measures to mitigate jetlag

8. DEPRESSION

EVERYTHING STARTED WITH MY DIVORCE

My insomnia is long standing. It started some years ago after my divorce. My husband came home late in the evening and told me "I want to divorce". I was not expecting it at all. My parents have a happy marriage for more than 40 years. In my family we do not divorce. Marriage is for life. It was a shock. He was cold, distant and determined. We divorced some months later and the kids stayed with me: two, a boy and a girl, with 9 and 13 years of age. Difficult age. They missed the father and blame me for that.

I had to reorganize life. My parents helped with the children. Money was not enough, and I had to work more and more, more than before.

I went to a psychiatrist got medication and some extra pounds, but the depression improved. The depression improved but the self-esteem not, neither the insomnia. I got it that day and it came to stay. It is my daily companion.

Every night I feel the hours going by, without any sleep, or any shadow of sleep. I organize then my daytime jobs. With great precision I must say, the problem is that sometimes my mind circles around and does not come out of a specific thought. But I also try to stop my thoughts, DO NOT THINK, I say to me. The result is not brilliant; I am always worried with something: the children, the work, the home, and my parents, who are becoming old and requiring more support.

I am still alone, but my "ex" married again. Life is not fair, nor just.

Often insomnia has these characteristics. They start with a specific trigger, in this case the divorce, but many other losses, life events or changes can have the same effect[140]. *They are perpetuated by the modifications that occur afterwards and by insomnia itself. Finally, they occur in a prone person, often an anxious or perfectionist personality. This is what is called the 3 P model, with* **P**recipitating, **P**erpetuating and **P**redisposing factors[141].

Therapy aims breaking the cycle, namely reducing the perpetuating and by the predisposing factors.

In many women divorces have a devastating effect. They were raised with the idea of "happy for ever" and reality shows things differently. At the post-divorce they take care of the children, work more, forget themselves, gain weight and forget all romance. But divorce is not the end of life and there are many pleasant ways to live afterwards. Self-esteem must be raised, and deleterious habits and beliefs changed.

Furthermore, insomnia itself works as a perpetuating factor, with nocturnal rumination, and a negative conditioned response to what leads to a good sleep.

The risk of depression is high[142]. The mutual relations between insomnia and depression led to the term of "co-morbid" diseases. What can be treated and the other remains, as in this woman.

Handling effectively insomnia is therefore crucial. For the present time the first line treatment is cognitive behaviour therapy.

Do you feel low in mood and in life?

Seek help! Whenever a door is closed a window opens!

---

[140] Reffi AN, Kalmbach DA, Cheng P, Drake CL. The sleep response to stress: how sleep reactivity can help us prevent insomnia and promote resilience to trauma. J Sleep Res. 2023 Dec;32(6):e13892. doi: 10.1111/jsr.13892. Epub 2023 Apr 5. PMID: 37020247.

[141] Paul AM, Salas RE. Insomnia. Prim Care. 2024 Jun;51(2):299-310. doi: 10.1016/j.pop.2024.02.002. Epub 2024 Mar 13. PMID: 38692776.

[142] Benca RM, Peterson MJ. Insomnia and depression. Sleep Med. 2008 Sep;9 Suppl 1:S3-9. doi: 10.1016/S1389-9457(08)70010-8. PMID: 18929317.

9. SEXUAL LIFE IMPACT AND PROBLEMS

MY SEXUAL LIFE IS NOT GOING WELL

I don't sleep well.

I go to bed and sleep flies away.

I think about everything, what has happened this day, what will happen tomorrow

I have lots of worries, my mother who lives alone, my husband whose job is in risk, my own job and my chief's humour, my mother-in-law with the onset of an incipient dementia ...

I turn around, left to right, to supine, without finding position and sleep not coming.

Am I depressed? Yes, a little

All these worries upon my shoulders. My husband doesn't care, "everything will turn alright" he says, he is an optimist, dramas are not for him, but sometimes I can't stand his voice ... his touch ...

Yes, you know, sexual life is not going well. I have no desire, no pleasure, no willingness

I must stand my husband wishes, but I am relieved when it is finished.

Sometimes it even hurts ...

It was not always like that, the first years of our marriage it was OK, I enjoyed sex, but after my first son was born satisfaction reduced, and nowadays is null.

My sexual life is not going well ...

Sleep deprivation among men and women is reported as one of the causes of infertility. Sleep deprivation and circadian desynchrony generate stressful stimuli increasing the activation of

the Hypothalamus-Pituitary Adrenal (HPA) axis, and consequently, the production of corticosterone.

In men high corticosteroids result in a reduction of testosterone. In women it results in reduced gonadotropin and sex steroid secretion which lead to female infertility. In shift work women melatonin is also reduced[143].

Severity of sleep problems correlated with unstimulated arousal only in the male and female groups with higher Testosterone levels, but not in females with normal testosterone or taking anticontraceptive. Poorer sleep quality was associated with female dissatisfaction with sex life, and mostly in women with lower Testosterone levels[144]

Women have higher prevalence of both sexual and sleep dysfunction and worse sleep quality.

A Spanish study involving 975 adult women, showed that, in women, global sexual dysfunction (desire, excitation, anticipatory anxiety, level of sexual communication, satisfaction of sexual activity, previous caesarean) was associated with poorer sleep quality. Other factors associated to poor sleep quality were obesity, age, mental health problem, and musculoskeletal conditions[145].

In USA a study in 3433 menopausal women 75% had poor sleep quality, and 54% sexual dysfunction; sleep quality, but not sleep duration, was associated with sexual dysfunction[146].

[143] Lateef OM, Akintubosun MO. Sleep and Reproductive Health. J Circadian Rhythms. 2020 Mar 23; 18:1. doi: 10.5334/jcr.190. PMID: 32256630; PMCID: PMC7101004

[144] Costa R, Costa D, Pestana J. Subjective sleep quality, unstimulated sexual arousal, and sexual frequency. Sleep Sci. 2017 Oct-Dec;10(4):147-153. doi: 10.5935/1984-0063.20170026. PMID: 29410746; PMCID: PMC5760048.

[145] Martínez Vázquez S, Hernández Martínez A, Peinado Molina RA, Martínez Galiano JM. Association between sexual function in women and sleep quality. Front Med (Lausanne). 2023 Aug 10;10:1196540. doi: 10.3389/fmed.2023.1196540. PMID: 37636576; PMCID: PMC10457145.

[146] Kling JM, Kapoor E, Mara K, Faubion SS. Associations of sleep and female sexual function: good sleep quality matters. Menopause. 2021 Apr19;28(6):619-625. doi: 10.1097/GME.0000000000001744. PMID: 33878089.

In Turkey, in a group of women with fibromyalgia (FM) identical correlations were found between sexual dysfunction and poor sleep quality[147]. Other factors may however contribute to sexual dysfunction in FM, namely, stiffness, fatigue, depression and anxiety, sleep disorders, body image, premorbid sexual functioning, life stress, coping abilities, sexual attractiveness, skills of the partner and a history of sexual abuse[148].

In the elderly, in UK, gender differences occur in the relations between sleep and sexual dysfunction[149].

In women: 1) Moderate odds ratio were found between sexual arousal and low sleep quality; 2) Low sleep quality was associated with increased odds of orgasmic difficulty; 3) No associations between sleep duration and problems with sexual function

In men: 1) Moderate sleep quality was associated with increased odds of erectile difficulties; 2) low sleep quality was <u>not associated</u> with increased odds of orgasmic difficulty; 3) Significant associations between sleep duration and problems with sexual function.

<u>Poor sleep quality higher sexual disfunction</u>

<u>Treat your sleep for better sexual life</u>

---

[147] Amasyali AS, Taştaban E, Amasyali SY, Turan Y, Kazan E, Sari E, Erol B, Cengiz M, Erol H. Effects of low sleep quality on sexual function, in women with fibromyalgia. Int J Impot Res. 2016 Mar-Apr;28(2):46-9. doi:10.1038/ijir.2015.31. Epub 2015 Nov 19. PMID: 26581913.

[148] Bazzichi L, Giacomelli C, Rossi A, Sernissi F, Scarpellini P, Consensi A, Bombardieri S. Fibromyalgia and sexual problems. Reumatismo. 2012 Sep 28;64(4):261-7. doi: 10.4081/reumatismo.2012.261. PMID: 23024970.

[149] Smith L, Grabovac I, Veronese N, Soysal P, Isik AT, Stubbs B, Yang L, Jackson SE. Sleep Quality, Duration, and Associated Sexual Function at Older Age: Findings from the English Longitudinal Study of Ageing. J Sex Med. 2019 Mar;16(3):427-433. doi: 10.1016/j.jsxm.2019.01.005. Epub 2019 Feb 14. PMID: 30773496.

10. Marital risks

MY MARRIAGE IS BROKEN. I CAN'T HANDLE SHIFTS

"I can't sleep neither during the day nor during the night.

I used to do shift work calmly. I had no problems for 20 years.

I would work at night and sleep during the day. I would work during the day and sleep at night. It was simple!

I used to sleep when I needed to, sometimes more, sometimes less, but everything was fine.

Now it's a mess, both during the day and at night.

They gave me some pills to sleep but they did not do the trick."

"What were your shifts like?"

"Six days on during the day and six days on at night, then six days on in the afternoon, but as they changed it wasn't always like that."

"Why six days — it doesn't form a weekly routine."

"No, it doesn't, but it was like that, and I was always fine with it."

"What did you do?"

"I was a production controller. The factory cannot stop."

"Do you smoke?"

"Yes, 2 packets a day."

"Do you take sleeping pills?"

"Yes, I take various, Dormonoct, Xanax, Lexotan."

"Do you tend to be anxious or irritable?"

"A little."

"Have you ever had any accidents?"

"No. I mean once I was so lucky I didn't die. I was coming from the night shift and left the road. It was a field that had been seeded. Luckily the car stopped in the middle of the potato field and did not hit anything. I needed a breakdown van to get me out of there. I hadn't even remembered that anymore. Another thing, Doctor, is that I am very forgetful!

I forget what I am going to do. The other day I couldn't remember my cashpoint "pin". I didn't remember it was my wife's birthday. It was awful!... But it wasn't my fault. It seems that things just get swept out of my memory."

"Do you tend to be depressed?"

"Yes. I don't feel like doing anything. My wife complains and things are going badly at home. Yes, that's also going badly, and I don't feel like doing anything, anything... There was a time when we spent weeks without seeing each other. She went to work, and I went to sleep. When she got home, I went to work. It wasn't very nice.

The marriage is broken, she asked me the divorce some days ago

Spending my days and nights without sleeping is horrible. I'm 45 years old and I'm an old man!

I don't know what to do"

There are people who can handle shift work better; generally, "night owls" can handle it better than "morning larks". There are those who can handle it for years without any problems, but around 40 – 45 years of age they start to be unable to continue to put up with it.

Shift work leads to greater risks of:

- *Depression.*
- *Marriage problems.*
- *Headaches.*
- *Memory complaints.*
- *Greater consumption of tobacco and/or drugs.*
- *Greater consumption of sleeping pills.*
- *Greater risks of road accidents.*

Shifts have organized scheduled routines.

- *You shouldn't function backwards in time, that is "night-afternoon", but rather forwards: "afternoon – night".*
- *You should adjust yourself to a weekly rhythm of 7 days.*
- *You shouldn't do more than 5 shifts of 8 hours a week.*
- *Or more than 4 of 12 hours.*
- *The shift should never start before 7:00.*
- *There should be rest intervals.*

What is more, having excessive daily work, excessive work at the weekends and carrying out duties where there is no means of taking decisions is equally likely to worsen the problem of working shifts.

Prophylactic naps before a night shift are also very effective.

When returning from a night shift, workers should avoid exposing themselves to light (wear dark glasses, for example) and should avoid driving.

Shift work reduces total sleep time.

There are people who should not work shifts, specifically those who have a sleep pathology, who suffer from a psychiatric disease, a sleep disorder, alcohol and drug abuse, patients with epilepsy, diabetes or heart disease.

Marital problems in shift work, excessive work, late and irregular schedules have three main causes: 1) The irregularity of encounters between spouses and the allowance this irregularity offers, bilaterally, to infidelity excuses; 2) Sleep deprivation with the associated libido reduction and lower sexual hormones production; 3) Fatigue and depression; 4) Marital discussions: "Never there", "Always tired", "Nothing you do is right"; 5) The negative sexual impact of medication.

In men reduction in testosterone is clear and leads to erectile dysfunction (ED), decreased libido, loss of pubic and body hair, impaired orgasmic and ejaculatory function[150].

The sleep disorders with high prevalence of sexual dysfunctions are: 1) Obstructive sleep apnea, in which the incidence of ED among male, ranges from 47.1% to 80.0%; 2) Insomnia and chronic sleep insufficiency, in which sexual dysfunction is more common among older men and menopausal women; 3) Circadian disorder among which shift work; 4) Sleep related movement disorders: although the prevalence of sexual dysfunction is not known in restless legs syndrome and in periodic leg movements (PLM) the PLM prevalence is very high in patients with sexual dysfunction5) hypersomnias and parasomnias the prevalence of sexual dysfunction is not known

Are you in a shift work job? Take great care!

---

[150] Cho JW, Duffy JF. Sleep, Sleep Disorders, and Sexual Dysfunction. World J Mens Health. 2019 Sep;37(3):261-275. doi: 10.5534/wjmh.180045. Epub 2018 Aug 14. PMID: 30209897; PMCID: PMC6704301.

F. Sleep Stories

1. FALLING ASLEEP AND WAKING UP

Sleep and wakefulness are two different states of our body and mind, regulated by different regions of the brain and by specific imbalances of neurotransmitters.

They influence each other, but to be fully awake sleep must be stopped, and to fall asleep wakefulness must be inhibited.

Falling asleep and waking up are not on-off phenomena, so one cannot neither fall asleep nor wake up as if you are pressing one on-off switch.

Thera are in both progressive changes in neurotransmitters, behaviour, **EEG**, muscle tonus, respiration, heart rate, which globally aim to prepare entrance in the next stage, be it awake or asleep.

These transitions between wakefulness and sleep are therefore special moments associated with some instability.

This enhances the probability of associated problems, as explained subsequently.

HERE COMES THE SANDMAN

"When I give classes in the morning, I can immediately see who is awake or sleepy. The sleepy students are pale and have bags under their eyes; they blink often, and you can see that they are not really hear what I am saying."

"I can hold on well and can sleep in classes without anyone realising."

"You?! You're an embarrassment. In 8am classes you do indeed sit up and sleep with your eyes open, but you went too far the other day. You started to nod off and slip off the chair. I caught you halfway because the Teacher was looking at you with beady eyes. Only snoring was missing!"

"When I was in the army I managed to nap while on parade. Sometimes I wavered a little, but I had everything well worked out."

"My husband is impossible. He falls asleep while he is talking to me. He stops replying and 'shuts off'."

"I can tell when my son is about to fall asleep, because he starts to bat his eyelids, yawns, nods off, blinks more rapidly, breathes more slowly and stops replying to what I am saying. After sleeping, whether sitting down or in bed, he snores a little."

"As for me, when I am really falling asleep, all my body twitches. It seems as if I am going to fall down and I wake up startled. It happens mostly when I am tired. Recently it has been more frequent, because I am preparing for the basketball championship and training several hours a day."

"That happened to me too. Several times in fact! Besides the feeling of falling, it seems that I sometimes see a light."

"My little son has that too. It seems as if all his body is convulsing."

These descriptions are of phenomena associated with falling asleep.

1) *Increased blinking.*

2) *Yawning, in animals (mammals, birds, reptiles) and humans, occurs before falling asleep, in tiredness and in monotonous situations. Yawning is "contagious" as it has a social synchronisation effect.*

3) *There is a reduction in muscle tone, mainly in the neck, which makes people to nod off.*

4) *Reaction to external stimuli diminishes and there are evident lapses in replies.*

5) *Closing your eyes implies light sleep. During this period there are slow movements of the eyes, which are impossible to imitate in wakefulness, and the EEG becomes slower, around 4 to 6 cycles per second (in vigilance this is greater than 10 cycles per second or even higher).*

6) *Breathing becomes more regular, and you can indeed snore a little, or breathe more deeply and slow.*

7) *There is a reduction in muscle tone in all muscles, and so it is difficult to remain standing.*

8) *The "twitches" when falling asleep are myoclonic jerks (hypnagogic jerks) and in most cases do not have clinical importance.*

9) *During this transition from wake to sleep rhythmic oscillations in the prefrontal cortex provide oscillatory entrainment of global cortical networks[151].*

The "Sandman" really does weigh on the eyelids.

---

[151] Sakata S, Yamamori T, Sakurai Y. 7-12 Hz cortical oscillations: behavioral context and dynamics of prefrontal neuronal ensembles. Neuroscience. 2005;134(4):1099-111. doi: 10.1016/j.neuroscience.2005.05.018. PMID: 16019153.

I FALL DOWN AT SLEEP ONSET

When I am about to fall asleep, I jump, as if I was having a startle and have the feeling of falling down. It is somewhat frightening, and I wake up. Sometimes I hear a sound, or I have some vague images in front of me; nothing clear, what is really clear is the body jumping alone and waking me up.

Some days ago, it happened in succession, falling asleep, jumping, falling asleep, jumping and until I finally slept. I was too tired: the exams, the football match, the victory party, my only wish was to sleep and these falling down sensations prevented me to.

These events are called hypnic jerks[152,153] or hypnagogic myoclonus. They are usually not important, since they represent a sudden decrease in muscle tone, which, as it is too fast, leads to awakening. Therefore, they are more frequent in association with tiredness.

They are very common most people will have experienced them.

They are caused by the fact that when you are tired, the reduction in muscle tone in falling asleep is more rapid and you wake up with the falling sensation. They can be linked to small sensory phenomena, such as a light sensation, etc.

Usually they do not repeat, but in some rare patients they can occur in succession during sleep onset, preventing sleep and leading to worries and eventually insomnia. They should be investigated and treated. Convulsions or paroxysmal jerks during sleep onset should also be investigated.

Hypnic jerks occurs mostly whenever you are tired. Don't worry.

---

152 Walters AS. Clinical identification of the simple sleep-related movement disorders. Chest. 2007 Apr;131(4):1260-6. doi: 10.1378/chest.06-1602. PMID: 17426241.
153 Baldelli L, Provini F. Fragmentary Hypnic Myoclonus and Other Isolated Motor Phenomena of Sleep. Sleep Med Clin. 2021 Jun;16(2):349-361. doi: 10.1016/j.jsmc.2021.02.008. Epub 2021 Apr 15. PMID: 33985659.

A MONSTER VISITS MY ROOM OR MY SLEEP

— You know the initial phase of my sleep is quite complicated. Often there is a monster like image sitting at my bed and looking at me. In some days I can identify the eyes and the mouth, but usually is quite vague: a monster like appearance without a face. I already tried to speak with it, several times,

— What did you say?

— Well, I asked him what he was doing there and what did he want from me

— Did you get any answer?

— No, indeed ... no answer

— What do you think it is?

— Well, I don't know ...

— Do you believe it is real?

— Humm, well, I am uncertain

— Why? Are you frightened?

— It is..., it may be ... some paranormal effect or someone trying to speak with me ... You know my grandmother is a medium, so I believe ..., let's say in the family we believe these things are real ...I am afraid, yes! I am!

— Well, probably these visions are linked to your other complaints, your sleepiness, your falls, etc. I will explain that to you so that you are no longer afraid.

These feelings are called hypnagogic hallucinations or complex sleep related hallucinations[154]. Hypnagogic is anything that occurs at sleep onset. Hallucinations are unreal visions or sensations, considered as real by the person who has them.

---

154   Waters F, Ling I, Azimi S, Blom JD. Sleep-Related Hallucinations. Sleep Med Clin. 2024 Mar;19(1):143-157. doi: 10.1016/j.jsmc.2023.10.008. Epub 2023 Nov 29. PMID: 38368061.

These hallucinations are not a psychiatric symptom, neither a paranormal manifestation. They can have several modalities: visual, auditory, somesthesis (something touching the body), etc. or they can even represent complex plots, like someone around, a thief entering the house, etc. This means they are multimodal.

They can occur at sleep onset (more common) or upon awakening: they are then called hypnopompic.

They are a feature of narcolepsy[155], in which sleepiness and eventual sudden falls without conscience loss do exist.

Strange sensations or visions at sleep onset require a clinical diagnosis.

---

[155] Slowik JM, Collen JF, Yow AG. Narcolepsy. 2023 Jun 12. In: StatPearls [Internet]. Treasure Island (FL): StatPearls Publishing; 2024 Jan–. PMID: 29083681.

I HAVE SOME STRANGE FITS AT SLEEP ONSET

— Soon after falling asleep strange things do occur. My arm extends and I look to other side, sometimes also the leg. Occasionally I lost consciousness. Which side? I don't know exactly; may be the left.

— It is to the left; I am sure, due to our places in the bed. But you know, even when he does not lose consciousness, he is often a bit confused, and may say or vocalize some incomprehensible sounds.

— So far, I tried several treatments but without success. They mostly occur during sleep, or even at sleep onset.

— Well, the symptoms you describe look like seizures, therefore it is important to know several features: the age of onset, the frequency of occurrence, the precise temporal relation with sleep and its occurrence during awake or later in the night, previous diseases and familiar history and mostly which are the possible triggers and eventual associated neurological symptoms.

Epilepsy and sleep have close interconnections[156]; about one third of the epileptic patients have their seizures only during sleep, others have both during wakefulness and during sleep and others only during wakefulness.

Epilepsy can fragment sleep and can change sleep architecture, with decreased sleep efficiency and REM sleep, increased wakefulness, sleep stage shifts, arousals and fragmentation, while both epilepsy and epilepsy therapies can influence sleep and produce sleep symptoms, such as hypersomnia, insomnia and postictal hypersomnolence

---

[156] Kataria L, Vaughn BV. Sleep and Epilepsy. Sleep Med Clin. 2016 Mar;11(1):25-38. doi: 10.1016/j.jsmc.2015.10.008. Epub 2016 Jan 9. PMID: 26972031.

In sleep related epilepsies the occurrence is either at sleep onset, across the night during **NREM** sleep and upon awakening.

Sleep, mostly **NREM** sleep stages, promotes epileptic seizures due to the synchronized effect upon neuronal populations. This synchronization effect facilitates the occurrence of interictal discharges, and the spread of epileptic discharges and therefore epileptic seizures in prone patients. Furthermore, the instability of sleep initiation increases the risk of the paroxysmal epileptic activity. In opposite direction **REM** sleep inhibits interictal activity but some sleep disorders, such as, sleep apnoea, may increase epileptic seizures probability

Epileptic events can be distinguished from other paroxysmal events by the stereotypic movements, the presence of interictal paroxysmic activity, the duration of minutes, the temporal occurrence along all night, the possibility of repetition twice or more times in one night.

The behaviour of epileptic seizures may vary a lot, from the motor seizure described in the above story to complex motor behaviours, dreams, etc.

Typical examples are **ADNFLE (Autosomal Dominant Nocturnal Frontal Lobe Epilepsy)** more recently called **Autosomal Dominant Sleep-Related Hypermotor (Hyperkinetic) Epilepsy**[157], **Benign childhood epilepsy with centrotemporal spikes (BECTS), nocturnal childhood occipital epilepsy (Panayiotopoulos Syndrome), Juvenile myoclonic epilepsy, Primary generalized seizures on awakening, Epilepsy with continuous spike and wave, Landau Kleffner syndrome.** Furthermore, in temporal lobe epilepsy

---

[157] Kurahashi H, Hirose S. Autosomal Dominant Sleep-Related Hypermotor (Hyperkinetic) Epilepsy. 2002 May 16 [Updated 2023 Mar 23]. In: Adam MP, Feldman J, Mirzaa GM, et al., editors. GeneReviews® [Internet]. Seattle (WA): University of Washington, Seattle; 1993-2024. Available from: https://www.ncbi. nlm.nih.gov/books/NBK1169/

MY SLEEP AND I

complex phenomena may occur, such as recurrent nightmares, hallucinations and dejá vu.

Diagnosis implies detailed history, neurologic examination, nocturnal video-polysomnography with **21 EEG** electrodes and imaging techniques to detect structural brain abnormalities.

The seizures should and must be treated adequately, to achieve whenever possible, their complete remission.

Walking during your sleep is not necessarily sleepwalking.

Strange fits or bizarre behaviours require both diagnosis and treatment.

WAKING UP IS REALLY DIFFICULT

Susan: I sleep 8 hours a night, but waking up is a problem. I drag myself between the kitchen, the bedroom and the bathroom.

Sophie: I wake up as fresh and restored. I get up in a trice and get on without any major problems. I am in good spirits and fully awake.

Susan: I spill the coffee. I trip up on the rugs. I even bump into the doors. And nobody dare talk to me. My mood would cut a knife in two. Don't speak to me, or the answer will be rude. My mum gets so angry about the way I reply. She says that sometimes I grunt and other times I mutter something, but the most usual answer is very cutting. Give it half an hour and everything is fine.

Charlotte: Well, I am different from both of you. I wake up, then I like to stay a little bit in bed just doing nothing special, then I get up and do my things.

Moving from sleep to wakefulness is not immediate. Sleep has its own "inertia"[158], which means you do not wake up just like that.

There is in fact a period of transition, which for some people can be as much as 30 or 60 minutes, where the inertia of sleep shows itself through slow reactions, uncoordinated gestures and a bad mood.

Sleep inertia in terms of survival seems disadvantageous since whenever the need of sudden awake is needed, sleep inertia counteracts the need of a well working brain.

However, there are two aspects to consider. One relates to the Three process model of Sleep regulation which includes the Process S (SLEEP), the Process C (CIRCADIAN), the Process W

---

[158] Hilditch CJ, McHill AW. Sleep inertia: current insights. Nat Sci Sleep. 2019 Aug 22;11:155-165. doi: 10.2147/NSS.S188911. PMID: 31692489; PMCID: PMC6710480.

(WAKE); in this model Sleep Inertia at sleep offset at counteracts the low homeostatic drive for sleep and the rising circadian drive for wakefulness, balancing both. The other view is the "universal" functional organization of physiological processes, for which sudden changes are, in principle dangerous.

During this transition period answers may not be very suitable and there may be temporary memory problems: you cannot provide names, remember a telephone number, etc.

Sleep inertia problems are particularly important in shift workers who nap during their shift. When waking up suddenly they may not be able to provide an adjusted reply with consequent problems.

This can also happen to those who sleep less than they need and suffer the effects of sleep deprivation. There is a "fight" between the sleep which they should have had and their present wakefulness.

As with other parameters, the sleep inertia varies greatly among individuals, being less for some, who wake up bright and breezy, and greater for others who wake up duller. Others include their inertia period in their normal activities and unknowingly hope that it has gone away by the time they get up.

When waking up in the morning, there are transition "gray zones" between sleep and wakefulness.

I CANNOT MOVE UPON AWAKENING

I am going to tell you something that is worrying me. I wake up in the middle of the night or early morning and I cannot move.

It is just like being paralysed, but I am certain that I am not dreaming. It's just that I cannot move. This happens two or three times a month, mostly when I am either not sleeping much or sleeping in, in the morning. When it happens, I get a bit scared and afraid that something has happened to me. It is a weird and unpleasant feeling. If for example I had to quickly run away I know I would not be able to, and that scares me a lot.

There is nothing else wrong. I sleep well, and I don't fall asleep during the day. I don't snore. I have never fainted. I don't have insomnia, and I don't have any bouts of depression. I practise gymnastics regularly and go swimming at the weekends. I do not stay up all night and I get good marks at the university.

This is probably a sleep paralysis, which is explained by the fact that REM sleep atonia (that is, the absence of muscle tone), persists into wakefulness, in the transition between wakefulness and sleep.

As an isolated symptom it is not especially important, or requiring of treatment, but it can form part of the four main symptoms of Narcolepsy.

It can be linked to hypnagogic hallucinations, visions on falling asleep, and the situation is then extremely frightening for the patient. The hallucinations may include an intruder or being associated with the feeling of pressure upon the thorax (incubus type)[159].

---

[159] Farooq M, Anjum F. Sleep Paralysis. 2023 Sep 4. In: StatPearls [Internet]. Treasure Island (FL): StatPearls Publishing; 2024 Jan–. PMID: 32965993.

Predisposing factors include sleep deprivation, irregular sleep-wake schedules, and jetlag[160].

In a systematic review the factors associated with sleep paralysis were substance use, stress, panic disorder, trauma (post-traumatic stress disorder), genetic influences, physical illness, personality, intelligence, anomalous beliefs, sleep problems, symptoms of psychiatric illness and anxiety symptoms[161].

From a cultural point of view, in many cultures sleep paralysis has been interpreted as the action of a bad force (spirit, Shaman, witch), which either puts pressure on sleepers' chests and prevents them from moving, or possesses their spirit with some malignant intention. Many cases of kidnapping by extra-terrestrials in the United States match descriptions of sleep paralysis.

Even in western culture, sleep paralysis is interpreted as an esoteric experience by some patients who feel that the paralysis is linked to a sensory experience.

Sleep paralysis has physiological explanations; it does not need to be accounted for by esoteric causes.

[160] Stefani A, Högl B. Nightmare Disorder and Isolated Sleep Paralysis. Neurotherapeutics. 2021 Jan;18(1):100-106. doi: 10.1007/s13311-020-00966-8. Epub 2020 Nov 23. PMID: 33230689; PMCID: PMC8116464.
[161] Denis D, French CC, Gregory AM. A systematic review of variables associated with sleep paralysis. Sleep Med Rev. 2018 Apr;38:141-157. doi: 10.1016/j.smrv.2017.05.005. Epub 2017 Jun 8. PMID: 28735779.

HE SEEMS A BAD CONTROLLED ROBOT

— My son says that I exaggerate and that he is completely well, only a bit sleepy in the morning.

— Yes it is true, she always exaggerate and describes things and facts with a dimension that they don't have.

— Well, let's see. I must say in fact that, upon awakening, he does not behave normally, he goes against anything, tables, chairs, furniture and walls and if something is pushing him out of a normal behavioural procedure, it drops anything he has in his hands and is unable to handle the milk glass. Everything the napkins or towels are flooded with milk or any other liquid he is taking. He is like a jerky robot.

— This happens when I am tired and sleep less, not always.

— No Doctor this is increased when he is tired but happens quite often, even when he is not completely tired. Furthermore, some days ago you fainted in school and, of course, I am quite concerned

— They told me this is confusional arousals, or the sleep inertia or whatever it is.

— Well, I think it is better you do an EEG with both sleep and awakening recording, and then we discuss all matters with you. It is very likely something different from what you were told.

This boy has very likely juvenile myoclonic epilepsy (JME), which occurs mostly during awakenings or soon after them. Instead of the classical seizures the epileptic fits are mostly myoclonia, ie, jerks of the upper limbs with clumsiness or dropping of objects, or of all the body inducing a marked instability of posture and gestures leading to jerky and brisk movements, seemingly like the old robots. Absences and generalized tonic-clonic seizures (convulsions) might also occur.

The EEG is quite characteristic with generalized paroxysmal activity of polyspike and waves, often coincident with the jerks; an abnormal response to photic stimulation is common.

Besides occurrence after awakening from nocturnal sleep or from a nap, usually 30 to 60 minutes after it. Despite the morning occurrence there are no consistent links with Chronotype, but patients JME have significant alterations in sleep architecture and decline in the quality of sleep[162].

JME seizures are triggered by sleep deprivation, stress, fatigue, alcohol intake; mental or emotional stress may also be triggers, as well as photic stimuli, from stroboscopic light, discos, computer games, etc.

Some cases of JME are hereditary. The EEG is mandatory and crucial for diagnosis, since imaging brain tests are usually normal. Treatment by adequate specialists (neurologists, epileptologists) is mandatory, since adequate medication is efficient in 90% of them.

Clumsiness upon awakening in adolescents must be taken seriously

---

[162] Xu L, Guo D, Liu YY, Qiao DD, Ye JY, Xue R. Juvenile myoclonic epilepsy and sleep. Epilepsy Behav. 2018 Mar;80:326-330. doi: 10.1016/j.yebeh.2017.11.008. Epub 2018 Jan 19. PMID: 29358100.

2. SLEEPING TOO LITTLE AND SLEEPING BADLY

Insomnia is the most prevalent sleep complaint

There are serious health risks for chronic insomnia.

The large number and the marked diversity of insomnia precipitating factors and comorbidities introduces in the insomnia spectrum a significant variability, so that, we must say "There are not two equal insomnias!"

Treatment, as Judith Owens says, implies accurate knowledge of the eventual multiple causes.

"Insomnia is an indication, not a chaos. It's like an ache. You're not going to provide a patient ache medicine without figuring out what's reasoning the pain." — Judith Owens

I STAY UP ALL NIGHT

I do not know how I can withstand not sleeping for so long!

Since several months ago I do not sleep at all, never mind the many years where I have slept badly.

Pills do nothing for me. I have taken everything... pills from my GP, who gave me alprazolam, the hypertension doctor who gave me Loprazolam[163], and the Psychiatrist who prescribed Cyamemazine[164], and so many more...

Nothing has had any effect. Nothing!

I still take Lorazepam... I have been doing so for years.... I do not know who first prescribed it for me.

At first it had an effect, but now it seems like some little devil gets hold of my eyelids and won't let me close them.

The hours pass. Falling asleep is a punishment, it means tossing and turning in bed, and then I wake up just two hours later.

Watching the hours pass - 3:00 am, 4:00 am! So little time left to sleep...

It is almost morning. I must go to work and how can I go without sleeping?

I have so many bags under my eyes. Beauty sleep? No way!

Yesterday I slept on the sofa watching television – the programmes suck but I just cannot sleep in my bed. The bed is lumpy.

Tomorrow morning I'll be up.

---

[163] Loprazolam has as brand names: Dormonoct, Havlane, Sonin, Somnovit
[164] Cyamemazine has as brand name Tercian

Waking up the kids, getting them washed, having breakfast and getting ready for school.

John is always a nightmare, dragging himself from chair to chair with his eyes closed, half awake half asleep. Maria is speedier.

Since John was born, I haven't been able to sleep. He wouldn't let me sleep. He was an impossible child and purely and simply would not sleep. At night he wanted to play and during the day he still did not sleep. He wasn't a normal child!

Until then I used to sleep well but since he was born, I have stopped sleeping.

I cannot forget that I must buy some rice and milk, and there also is no fruit or wool detergent.

So much to do... How am I going to endure this?

The boss has been unbearable. Today he wanted the mock-ups of the labels ready, when he asked for them just yesterday. I should have told him to take a hike!

"Gloria, I want this stuff ready today. See if you can hurry it up!"

For today, how is that possible?! He just gave me the job yesterday!

"See if you can hurry it up!"

I am forty years old, and I have worked there for 20 years. Hurry it up, he says... can you believe that?!

I must sleep.

C'mon, stop thinking, see if you can calm down. This cannot be like this.

"See if you can hurry it up...", good grief, what a cheek, I've worked there for 20 years. I give it my best, and that's the thanks I get.

I am going to try and sleep, perhaps say the rosary.

Ave Maria, full of grace, the Lord is with thee … and if I do not sleep? Blessed is the fruit of thy womb… it's 5:00 am.

I must go to the bathroom. It's cold. I am going to drink a glass of water. I'll have a glass of water and take a Zolpidem[165].

It's so cold…

Shall I take 1 or 2?

I can't handle 2, because I will have a heavy head.

John is sleeping intrepidly. How happy for him. I can't make any noise.

I'll just take one pill.

The bed is still warm. Maybe I'll sleep now.

It's 5:30 am Oh, Lord.

"Hurry it up", he said.

I can't take so many pills.

……..

Next morning:

C'mon John, hurry up. You're going to be late. Don't answer back like that or you'll get a slap.

Naughty! Stupid! Irresponsible! You take hours to do anything.

I'm a bundle of nerves. I can't take it any longer.

Did I burn the toast?

It's your fault for not leaving me quiet.

---

[165] Zolpidem has as brand names: Ambien, Ambien CR, Intermezzo, Stilnox, Stilnoct, Sublinox, Hypnogen, Zonadin, Sanval, Zolsana and Zolfresh

Hurry up, Maria. Oh, you're ready!

Where are the car keys? Help me find the car keys!

Of course I'm tired.

I haven't slept and I have got up, had a shower, made the bed, woken you, got breakfast ready, screamed and now I can't find the car keys.

We're going to be late.

Did I have something to do for today? What was it? I'm so forgetful, am I suffering from Alzheimer's?

Your father is still fast asleep, and I have been rushing around.

Ah! I had to phone John's dentist. I mustn't forget.

Let's go. It's late now. Let's hope the car starts and there isn't much traffic.

C'mon. I'm waiting for you.

Don't be naughty!!!

Please, let's go...

This patient has chronic insomnia[166,167, 168]

---

[166] American Academy of Sleep Medicine. ICSD-3—International Classification of Sleep Disorders. American Academy of Sleep Medicine, Chicago, 2014

[167] Kaur H, Spurling BC, Bollu PC. Chronic Insomnia. [Updated 2023 Jul 10]. In: StatPearls [Internet]. Treasure Island (FL): StatPearls Publishing; 2024 Jan-. Available from: https://www.ncbi.nlm.nih.gov/books/NBK526136/

[168] Riemann D, Espie CA, Altena E, Arnardottir ES, Baglioni C, Bassetti CLA, Bastien C, Berzina N, Bjorvatn B, Dikeos D, Dolenc Groselj L, Ellis JG, Garcia-Borreguero D, Geoffroy PA, Gjerstad M, Gonçalves M, Hertenstein E, Hoedlmoser K, Hion T, Holzinger B, Janku K, Jansson-Fröjmark M, Järnefelt H, Jernelöv S, Jennum PJ, Khachatryan S, Krone L, Kyle SD, Lancee J, Leger D, Lupusor A, Marques DR, Nissen C, Palagini L, Paunio T, Perogamvros L, Pevernagie D, Schabus M, Shochat T, Szentkiralyi A, Van Someren E, van Straten A, Wichniak A, Verbraecken J, Spiegelhalder K. The European Insomnia Guideline: An update on the diagnosis and treatment of insomnia 2023. J Sleep Res. 2023 Dec;32(6):e14035. doi: 10.1111/jsr.14035. PMID: 38016484.

The patient has difficulty in initiating sleep, in maintaining sleep continuity, and has poor sleep quality, the symptoms occur for a long time (many years), i.e., more than 3 months and daily (more than 3 times per week (ICSD3).

Insomnia is the most prevalent sleep disorder in USA, circa 30% of the people, in Europe the prevalence is lower, around 10% of the adults.

In this case it is related to anxiety, depression, too many worries and responsibilities in her daily life.

The insomnia starts with a specific problem but then carries on getting worse due to life's events.

She must manage all the housework, bringing up the children and has an unrewarding job where she is not held in esteem.

She has a sleep-related attentional bias sleeping better in the sofa.

During the night introspection, worry, and rumination emerge.

She makes important efforts to sleep (praying, raising up, taking medication, glass of water, trying to calm down) and has arousing habits such as looking at the clock. She has recursive thoughts about the same event. Besides this, she is taking pills, which down the years have now become a habit.

Anxiety and depression are frequent insomnia comorbidities[167].

Furthermore, there is some eventual family insomnia history, with a sleepless son.

The genes associated with insomnia are Apolipoprotein (Apo) E4, PER3 4/4, HLA-DQB1*0602, homozygous Clock gene 3111C/C Clock and short (s-) allele of the 5-HTTLPR[166]. Family and twin studies confirm that chronic insomnia can have a genetic component *(heritability coefficients between 42% and 57%); research found an imbalance of sleep-wake regulation with overactivity of the arousal systems, hypoactivity of the sleep-inducing systems, or both[169].*

The arousing systems increase is multimodal: increase in beta activity spectral power during sleep; patients have a sleep-related attentional bias with increased cue-induced amygdala reactivity to sleep-related pictures; reduced deactivation of the default mode network which may be related with symptoms of introspection, worry, and rumination; cortisol elevation reflecting hypothalamic-pituitary-adrenal axis hyperactivity; and increased sympathetic activity reflected in studies of heart rate variability[168].

Moderate and severe insomnia is more frequent in women and the elderly.

The recommendations are cognitive behaviour therapy, to abolish the arousing cycle, she is in. First it is necessary for her to change her attitudes, the worries and problems in her life. She needs to reduce the number of tasks and have a more positive attitudes, avoiding turning everything into a drama, and share the tasks that she cannot handle alone. Her dependency on pills, anxiety and depression implies specific pharmacological thera[167].

Many celebrities have suffered from insomnia. Some of them can be mentioned, though it is not known exactly what type of insomnia they suffered from: Marlene Dietrich, Franz Kafka, Theodore Roosevelt, Judy Garland, Groucho Marx and Mark Twain.

---

[169] Riemann D, Nissen C, Palagini L, Otte A, Perlis ML, Spiegelhalder K. The neurobiology, investigation, and treatment of chronic insomnia. Lancet Neurol. 2015 May;14(5):547-58. doi: 10.1016/S1474-4422(15)00021-6. Epub 2015 Apr 12. PMID: 25895933.

Day and night mutually influence each other. A bad day leads to a bad night and vice versa.

Don't give up, everything has a solution and can be solved but never forget:

TAKE CARE OF YOUR SLEEP

I DON'T SLEEP SINCE MY BABY IS BORN

When I was young, I used to sleep very well. Many people envied me even, since I was a sound sleeper. It changed with my first baby. Insomnia started during pregnancy, but when he was born he didn't sleep, that is, he would sleep during the day and was awake at night.

My "Karma" started then. I was awake all night long and working during the day. My job was easier in what concerns schedules than my husband's work. He could be fired; I could arrive later, so I stayed awake all night long. The baby would cry, have is milk, crying for us, coming to our bed finally. And there I was tired, red eyes with dark circles, irritable, shouting at low threshold, depressed.

My relationship with my husband was impacted. I had no wish for anything, especially for … that … certainly. I want to sleep and to rest.

He started sleeping well, (well … it was never well) by the age of 5. It was then I got the second one. Second pregnancy, second delivery, second son! He does not sleep either. So, I am in despair. My tears fall, unwanted and unnoticed. The fatigue is no longer fatigue, it is an absolute exhaustion. I shout at the boys. I shout to my husband. I shout … I feel one day I will simply scream: a big and endless scream.

For many women events related to pregnancy, birth, a sick new-born, or a sleepless baby are the insomnia precipitating factor.

97% of the women does not sleep well during pregnancy; sleep impairment is a risk for increased inflammation, gestational diabetes, pre-eclampsia, postpartum depression, mood disorders[170].

---

[170]   Chaudhry SK, Susser LC. Considerations in Treating Insomnia During Pregnancy: A Literature Review. Psychosomatics. 2018 Jul-Aug;59(4):341-348. doi: 10.1016/j. psym.2018.03.009. Epub 2018 Mar 21. PMID: 29706359.

The subsequent needs of the new-born, namely feeding and caring, are clear perpetuating factors. The presence of post-partum depression may aggravate the clinical picture.

Care must be taken with other associated sleep disorders, namely, obstructive sleep apnea and restless legs syndrome (RLS).

Women often have sleep apnoea wit insomnia symptoms. During pregnancy the predisposing factors are increased BMI, increased age and hypertension. Mother risks are gestational diabetes, gestational hypertension, pre-eclampsia, cardiomyopathy, pulmonary embolism, higher likelihood to have a caesarean delivery or a preterm delivery. Baby risks are low birth weight and being small-for-gestational-age. CPAP treatment may be recommended[171].

The development or worsening of RLS in pregnancy accounts for hormonal fluctuations (increased levels of estrogen, progesterone, prolactin, and thyroid hormones may be linked with lower dopamine levels), iron, ferritin and folate metabolism, vitamin D deficiency, genetic factors, zinc and magnesium changes[172]; treatment implies usually supplementation of the associated deficiencies.

Treating pregnancy insomnia is a challenge due to the difficulties of using medication and their putative risks for the baby.

Non pharmacologic treatments should be started: sleep hygiene rules (stimulus control techniques, circadian regulation, fluid restriction, screen restriction, exercise, morning light exposure, etc), cognitive behaviour therapy.

---

[171] Tayade S, Toshniwal S. Obstructive Sleep Apnea in Pregnancy: A Narrative Review. Cureus. 2022 Oct 17;14(10):e30387. doi: 10.7759/cureus.30387. PMID: 36407139; PMCID: PMC9668203.

[172] Mendes A, Silva V. Possible etiologies of restless legs syndrome in pregnancy: a narrative review. Sleep Sci. 2022 Oct-Dec;15(4):471-479. doi: 10.5935/1984-0063.20220080. PMID: 36419819; PMCID: PMC9670777.

Pharmacologic treatments must consider the associated risks for the baby, the pregnancy trimester, the mother health status and risks.

A sick new-born is another worrying factor, which together with the fear that something might happen to the child perpetuates and reinforces insomnia

A sleepless baby is a serious event in a woman, and in a couple's life. Often it is considered as a "must", something she will have to stand and overcome. Often, but not necessarily always, the problem is triggered by the first child.

A sleepless baby interferes with the parents as a couple; the required childcare becomes a priority, which by itself affects sleep.

Marked attention must be given to the couple harmony, since both are needed to take care of the child. This will not be done properly if both are exhausted.

However several aspects must be set clear: healthy babies sleep well, and their sleep is often troubled by their parents' behaviour; your healthy baby will sleep through the night and you don't need to survey all the baby movements; whenever taking care of the baby is a heavy burden ask for help and advice; father and mother should keep their intimacy throughout the growing of their baby; being hyper vigilant over your baby sleep is a big mistake; both parents and the baby deserve a good sleep to enjoy the pleasure of mother and fatherhood.

People who say they sleep like a baby usually don't have one. (Leo J. Burke)

I HAVE NO PROBLEMS FALLING ASLEEP, BUT I AWAKE UP OFTEN

I fell asleep in 15 to 20 minutes, without any problem. I am usually sufficiently tired at night, so sleep comes easily. It has always been like that. It is however difficult staying asleep and the exhaustion I feel upon my morning awakening is unbearable. M y head weights many ... many pounds, it hurts but the pain disappears sometime after I take a shower.

The mind is however not clear; it floats and drifts around until the second cup of coffee.

Dreams are strange. I forget them easily, but I dream more often nowadays. No nightmares, mostly dreams about common daily life. Nothing special

Awakening at night is boring, boring and tiring. I don't know what to do. I turn around a lot; my wife complains, I don't let her sleep. I look at the watch and see the time passing by with eyes wide open and no sleep. Nothing helps going to the WC, eating, working at the computer, TV, nothing.

No, I don't snore. Sometimes I feel something in my chest, but my heart is OK.

I am tired and sometimes sleepy during the day.

Waking up often represents what is called, a fragmented sleep. Sleep, both is REM and NREM is interrupted by brief and repetitive arousals or awakenings. This often prevents the deeper phases of sleep, and both N3 and REM are reduced, but the reduction upon the total sleep time is usually less impressive. Fatigue, headaches and sleepiness are frequent associated complaints

The increased number of arousals favours dreams, which are usually easily forgotten

- **The reason for this sleep fragmentation must be looked after, since the complaints is usually unspecific:**
- **Some patients snore and might have sleep apnoea (OSAS).**
- **Some might have what is called an upper airway resistance syndrome.**
- **Others might have periodic limb movements of sleep (PLMS).**
- **Some may have cardiac arrhythmias**
- **Others oesophageal reflux.**
- **Medical disorders may be a possible cause.**

Medical and neurological disorders that can be comorbid within insomnia are: cardiovascular disorders, diabetes mellitus, chronic kidney disorders, chronic obstructive pulmonary disorders, rheumatic disorders, chronic pain, malignant disorders, OSAS, RLS/ PLMS, neurodegenerative disorders, cerebrovascular disorders, traumatic head injury, fatal familiar insomnia[173].

Another cause may be excessive work and work stress; patients fell asleep since they are exhausted, but they wake at the middle of the night with daytime worries

In summary these patients must be thoroughly investigated and perform a polysomnography and treated accordingly.

In case you wake up many times per night, do not wait more. Ask for help

---

[173] Riemann D, Espie CA, Altena E, Arnardottir ES, Baglioni C, Bassetti CLA, Bastien C, Berzina N, Bjorvatn B, Dikeos D, Dolenc Groselj L, Ellis JG, Garcia-Borreguero D, et al. The European Insomnia Guideline: An update on the diagnosis and treatment of insomnia 2023. J Sleep Res. 2023 Dec;32(6):e14035. doi: 10.1111/ jsr.14035. PMID: 38016484.

I SLEEP 7 HOURS BUT I WAKE UP EXTREMELY TIRED

I sleep 7 hours a day, I have no difficulty to fall asleep and I do not wake during the night.

My sleep is quiet, I do not snore.

?!

All my answers are negative: No dreams, no screams, no kicks, no sweating, no nothing!

People say I sleep like a baby but in the morning, I am exhausted, as if a truck went over my body.

In some patient's sleep is not curtailed, apparently not disturbed but it has no restorative effect- Nonrestorative sleep (NRS).

In a review study the prevalence of NRS evaluated by yes-no questionnaire was 19.2-31.0% in men and 26.3-42.1% in women[174]; a multi-national survey using a telephone-based expert system showed a wide range of prevalence between countries, from 2.4% to 16.1% with the following question "How frequently are you bothered by the following problem: Your sleep is not refreshing, you don't feel rested even if the duration of your sleep is normal" [175].

The prevalence of NRS was higher in women and young subjects, in separated/divorced individuals, night shift workers, and subjects with 9 years or less of schooling, sleeping in a too stuffy bedroom and sleeping in an uncomfortable bed, smoking and alcohol taken at bedtime, physical illnesses, higher number of

---

[174] Matsumoto T, Chin K. Prevalence of sleep disturbances: Sleep disordered breathing, short sleep duration, and non-restorative sleep. Respir Investig. 2019 May;57(3):227-237. doi: 10.1016/j.resinv.2019.01.008. Epub 2019 Mar 1. PMID: 30827934.

[175] Ohayon, M. M. (2005). *Prevalence and Correlates of Nonrestorative Sleep Complaints. Archives of Internal Medicine, 165(1), 35*. doi:10.1001/archinte.165.1.35

medical consultations, long sleep duration, extra sleep time on weekends and/or days off, global sleep dissatisfaction, frequency of a bad night's sleep, mood disorders, physical fatigue or irritable mood, excessive daytime sleepiness, higher likelihood to take sleep medication[175].

The lack of this restorative effect may be due to several causes not apparent in the clinical evaluation, while observed in the polysomnography.

Among them is an increase in the amount of slow wave sleep. For reasons not yet clarified an increase in the homeostatic component of sleep results in tiredness, showing how important a correct balance among sleep stages is needed in other to achieve a restorative effect. In patients with Arousal Parasomnias and violent behaviours, this increase is a possible explanation for non-restorative sleep[176].

Another possibility is the presence of high frequency and small amplitude periodic limb movements of sleep, which are not observed by bed partners, and do not induce neither excessive dreaming nor headache, but are able to produce a superficial sleep with frequent microarousals.

Furthermore, sleep medication may induce an easy, quiet and bad quality sleep, with increased fast rhythms in the brain or increased number of spindles. Some medications may also induce a reduction in slow wave sleep, in REM sleep or in both. The same effect is shared by toxics as it is the case of alcoholic beverages, tobacco and drugs.

If you have a non-restorative sleep better look for its causes.

---

[176]   Mainieri G, Loddo G, Baldelli L, Montini A, Mondini S, Provini F. Violent and Complex Behaviors and Non-Restorative Sleep Are the Main Features of Disorders of Arousal in Adulthood: Real Picture or a More Severe Phenotype? J Clin Med. 2023 Jan 3;12(1):372. doi: 10.3390/jcm12010372. PMID: 36615171; PMCID: PMC9821298.

I WAKE IN THE MIDDLE OF THE NIGHT

I have no problems to fall asleep, but I wake up at the middle of the night, 2 or 3 hours after sleep onset.

It is annoying, since then I will remain asleep for several hours. At around 5am I will fall asleep again, but my sleep is curtailed, since I must wake at 7:30 am.

I don't understand what wakes me up.

In the beginning I used these moments as productive moments. I switched on the pc and started to develop my creative ideas.

Nowadays this is no longer possible. I get anxious with the few hours left to sleep and with the fact that I am sure I will not enter sleep easily.

I see some TV, go to the toilet, sometimes I eat something to calm down.

...

Yes, I become anxious in these moments and mostly tired. But I don't have any troublesome problem annoying me.

I must say that, sometimes, my mouth gets a strange burning flavour.

..

Yes, my dinner is usually late and heavy, since it is my single meal of the day. Lunch is vestigial, no free time then.

...

Yes it is heavy as far as quantity and quality are concerned. A good steak, swimming in a tasty sauce, with chips and no vegetables; cheese and some sweet as dessert.

...

I gained some weight, but my snoring is inconstant.

But my main problem, as I told you before, is to wake up at the middle of the night.

This is called middle term or intermediate insomnia. Waking up in the middle of the night is an unspecific symptom, which can be due to several problems.

Some people wake up and don't fall asleep again, others after waking up regain an interrupted sleep with frequent awakenings until the final morning awake, others after some time awake fall asleep again.

Some physiological and historical data are relevant to understand waking up in the middle of the night

After 4 or 5 hours of sleep, sleep pressure is highly reduced making difficult to fall asleep again.

Furthermore, historically, humans used to have the first and the second sleep, with an interval between both during which they prayed, eat, had sex, or meet the neighbours[177,178]. Descriptions appear for example in Charles Dickens' Barnaby Rudge (1840) and in Cervantes' D. Quixote (1605). The prayers schedules for Christian and Islamic religions also started/start at pre-dawn hours. Change occurred eventually during the industrial revolution and humans, to "spare" time, acquired the habit of a monophasic nocturnal sleep in adulthood.

---

[177] Roger A. Ekirch, 'Sleep We Have Lost: Pre-industrial Slumber in the British Isles', American Historical Review, 106 (2001), 343–386 (p. 344).

[178] Did we used to have two sleeps rather than one? Should we again? (theconversation.com)

This idea does not have universal agreement[179]; among the many arguments against concerning mostly data source and data interpretation, citation of a 2010 survey in which 31.2% of the general European population reported waking up at least three nights per week, and that 7.7% had difficulty resuming sleep[180] is used to refute the two sleeps. However, this could be seen as a perpetuation of old habits that in the present culture are not accepted.

Many people, nowadays, believe they must sleep in a single episode without awakening and get marked anxiety whenever they awake.

People can wake up because they have some concerns relative to existential events or circumstances.

People can wake up in the middle of the night because they have some medical problem which is enhanced by the lying position or by sleep itself.

Among those some deserve special reference: gastro-oesophageal reflux, sleep related arrhythmias, periodic limb movements of sleep, pain, asthma, sleep apnoea, poor adaptation to the CPAP machine[181], survivals of childhood abuse[182], etc.

---

[179] Boyce N. Have we lost sleep? A reconsideration of segmented sleep in early modern England. Med Hist. 2023 Apr;67(2):91-108. doi: 10.1017/mdh.2023.14. Epub 2023 Aug 1. PMID: 37525459; PMCID: PMC10404514.

[180] Ohayon MM. Nocturnal awakenings and difficulty resuming sleep: their burden in the European general population. J Psychosom Res. 2010 Dec;69(6):565-71. doi: 10.1016/j.jpsychores.2010.03.010. Epub 2010 Apr 28. PMID: 21109044.

[181] Caetano Mota P, Morais Cardoso S, Drummond M, Santos AC, Almeida J, Winck JC. Prevalence of new-onset insomnia in patients with obstructive sleep apnoea syndrome treated with nocturnal ventilatory support. Rev Port Pneumol. 2012 Jan-Feb;18(1):15-21. English, Portuguese. doi: 10.1016/j.rppneu.2011.06.016. Epub 2011 Nov 29. PMID: 22129574.

[182] Steine IM, Skogen JC, Krystal JH, Winje D, Milde AM, Grønli J, Nordhus IH, Bjorvatn B, Pallesen S. Insomnia symptom trajectories among adult survivors of childhood sexual abuse: A longitudinal study. Child Abuse Negl. 2019 Jul;93:263-276. doi: 10.1016/j.chiabu.2019.05.009. Epub 2019 May 23. PMID: 31129428.

In many cases, over this initial complaint, symptoms related to increased effort and to increased worries around the difficulty to fall asleep again may be present.

Reducing nocturnal awakening anxiety and a correct etiologic diagnosis are essential to start treatment.

Insomnia in the middle of the night has often organic causes

MY MOOD IS TERRIBLE

Brrr... another day, what a mess!

After a night with eyes wide open how can I start my day?

My life is a big mess.

I am not in the mood to come out of bed.

I do not have anybody to complain to.

I do not feel like going out, I do not feel able to work

I will stay in bed.

I have no energy to rise from bed.

My head is circling around, and I feel a dull headache

I will be dizzy if I came out of bed.

I am tired, so tired as if somebody took all energy from my body

Better not to live like that, alone, dizzy, without wishes, without pleasures

My shrink tells me I cannot stay in bed all day.

It is raining. It is sure that I will not leave my bed

The rain depresses me. It is as if the sky is crying on my pain

My pain is so deep and perfect as a cloister

My life is a big mess.

I am not in the mood to come out of bed.

I do not have anybody to complain to. I am alone.

I did not sleep more than 1 hour, altogether

I heard every hour at the tower clock

The rain is crying with me

My soul cries in pain and screams in fear

My life is martyrdom.

It is clear, that today, I will not work. The guy will certainly dismiss me this time.

My pain is deep and perfect as a middle age cloister.

With sharp squared angles pointed at my soul

They told me I would certainly sleep with this medication!

Brrr … I slept one hour.

I simply cannot sleep; I turn and turn and turn.

I try to be quiet, but something comes on my throat just to tighten it

If I do not sleep how I feel well?

My sleep is gone, my life is gone

No pleasures, no wishes, no wills

Better not to live like that, alone, dizzy and sad

"See other people," said my shrink. I don't like confusions, their noise annoys me, and their laughs are unbearable.

I have no solution, no aim.

I am sad and tired. How can I be well if don't sleep? How can I sleep if I am not well?

Nobody understands me, not even the shrink has the or patience to listen to me

"If you are not better, better change the medication"

I am good for nothing. My chest hurts, my throat is tightened by an invisible ball.

I am afraid of the night, turns and turns in bed, the sleep that does not come and these terrible thoughts.

Speaking with the dead, that is my night. My mother saying again and again: "You are good for nothing. Just look what you have done!" and my father not paying attention to me or to anything that might be at our home. The darkness of our home, the heavy curtains, the heavy furniture, the dubious light. "Don't open the window! I will get a cold"; "Be quiet or I will get a headache". My mother always shouting.

I have no solution, no objectives and no joy. Life sucks.

I will not have another day.

This case has symptoms of insomnia together with complaints of severe depression with sadness, desire to be isolated, difficulty in standing other people, tiredness, difficulty in handling daily tasks, somatic complaints, anguish, low self-esteem, negative thoughts focusing on people already passed away, possible childhood trauma, and suicidal ideation.

The association between insomnia and depression is complex, since they are considered co-morbid disorders. This means that insomnia can trigger a depression and depression can provoke insomnia, but the treatment of one of them does not assure that the other vanishes away.

Furthermore, this situation figures out the frequent presence of insomnia in psychiatric situations. The patient is depressed, and the fact she does not sleep increases the ideation negativity, establishing a vicious circle with reinforcement of negativity.

The relationship between sleep and depression may be explained by several mechanisms[183]*:*

- *Sleep loss may cause the elevation of cellular inflammation, with increased levels of inflammatory cytokines (IL-6 (interleukin 6) and TNF (tumour necrosis factor)) and these effects are more obvious in women. There is a strong relationship between inflammation and depression has also been observed and depressive patients have high levels of inflammatory markers*
- *Depression, mostly major depression, is associated with REM Sleep disturbances, mainly reduce REM sleep latency, increased number of REMs (rapid eye movements), long duration of the first REM episode. REM onset is determined by decrease in monoamines (serotonin [5-HT], norepinephrine [NE] and dopamine) and an increase in cholinergic activity (acetylcholine). In depression lower levels of monoamines are considered a main cause, and the basis for some pharmacologic treatments.*
- *Both depression and insomnia have proven genetic basis and consequent heritability.*
- *Furthermore, both depression and insomnia have, in some cases, circadian abnormalities*

Altogether these factors favour the joint occurrence

Patients with major depression have special abnormalities in the night sleep, namely, a reduced REM latency and an abnormal distribution of REM sleep in successive REM cycles. These abnormalities correlate with disease prognosis

---

[183] Fang H, Tu S, Sheng J, Shao A. Depression in sleep disturbance: A review on a bidirectional relationship, mechanisms and treatment. J Cell Mol Med. 2019 Apr;23(4):2324-2332. doi: 10.1111/jcmm.14170. Epub 2019 Feb 7. PMID: 30734486; PMCID: PMC6433686.

Patients with depression, in its different modalities, have usually a reduction of slow wave sleep and abnormalities in sleep microstructure.

Patients with comorbid insomnia and depression tend to suffer more severe depressive symptoms, longer durations of treatment and lower rates of remission

Treatment in the presented case, considering the suicidal ideation, must be quick and efficient. It usually implies medication with antidepressive medication, Cognitive Behaviour therapy, and psychotherapy. Deep brain stimulation may be useful in the treatment of resistant depression.

In the comorbid insomnia and depression the treatment of insomnia is usually quite relevant; CBT-I can improve sleep efficiency and achieve remission from insomnia[184].

Most psychiatric disorders are associated with insomnia.

---

[184] Wu JQ, Appleman ER, Salazar RD, Ong JC. Cognitive behavioral therapy for insomnia comorbid with psychiatric and medical conditions a meta-analysis. JAMA Intern Med. 2015;175(9):1461.

I HAVE NOT SLEPT SINCE I WAS A CHILD

I have never slept well. My mother used to tell me that as a child it was like a punishment for me to sleep. I didn't sleep very much, not even a nap and never wanted to go to bed. My mother did suffer as a result, poor thing!

How old was I? I don't know, around 4 or 5, or even less; I was very young.

Now it's the same. I don't sleep. I mean, I always sleep 4 to 5 hours and wake up tired. The smallest noise wakes me up at once. Even the sound of a fly... just a bit of buzzing and I wake up. It's a stupid thing to be so sensitive, isn't it? It's hard to fall asleep and I wake up amazingly easily.

My days are difficult. Something is missing ... not sure how to explain ... it is as if my body has not had its correct amount of rest and is lacking in a little energy.

Sleeping does not bring any pleasure. It's just a worry because I know it is going to go badly and so I try to avoid thinking about it.

I have tried everything; I have done everything to improve things. I don't drink coffee or anything like that. I mean, I don't smoke or drink. I go to bed around 10:30 or 11:00 pm I have a light dinner. When I go to bed I have a glass of milk or sometimes a special lime tea which somebody brought back for me from China. I don't watch television in bed, and I try not to think of anything, but it is difficult. I start thinking about work and life. Life is good, in fact... I like my job, I get on well with my husband, the children – I've got two – one of each – and they are good kids and do not give me any problems.

No, I don't overwork, but I like what I do and at work they like me. I am the personal assistant to the director. There is always a lot to do and I do everything, I organize everything. The work brings responsibility, and I don't like things badly done. My husband says that I am too organized and certainly I never stop — I am always doing something. I don't know what it means to sit on the sofa and do nothing. He tells me: "Sit here a little. Come on, stop, everything's done", but no, I can't. There's always something to do in the house! Yes, I am a perfectionist. I like things done well and I cannot stand disorganisation.

Nowadays I hardly take anything to sleep. It seems that pills just make things worse. I take Valerian which the doctor says is quite weak. I am afraid of becoming addicted and I do not like drugs. What is certain is that when I have taken a pill to sleep it sometimes even seems to have had the opposite effect. I had more insomnia, and the next day was worse.

I don't know if I can take this for many more years. This lack of sleep is slowly killing me. I don't get worse when there is a lot of stress, and I do not get better in the holidays. It always seems to be, more or less the same, for what it's worth. That is not to say that it doesn't get a bit worse when I have a problem, but my sleeping doesn't get much worse. It's the same in the holidays - when I can sleep I can't.

I am healthy. I have never had any major illnesses. I go to the gym twice a week, early in the morning because I know it is not good to work out at night.

My sleep hygiene is good, I think.

Nowadays childhood onset insomnia is included in the classification of chronic insomnia[185].

Insomnia with onset in childhood points to a constitutional dysfunction of the sleep-wakefulness system and /or to genetic causes.

---

[185] Sateia MJ. International classification of sleep disorders-third edition: highlights and modifications. Chest. 2014 Nov;146(5):1387-1394. doi: 10.1378/chest.14-0970. PMID: 25367475.

It starts early, often in the second decade of life.

Not everybody who has slept badly since childhood has this type of insomnia. Most of its causes are behavioural.

In contrast to other insomnia cases, there are no changes for the worse or the better in relation with the patient's life circumstances, and the level of complaint remains stable down through the years.

This is "insomnia" and not "short sleep" because it brings daily repercussions, like those of other insomnias, such as difficulties in concentrating, performance and memory, and lack of satisfaction with regard to sleep.

It has been shown that childhood onset insomnia and comorbid depression are less responsive to the treatments than are those with adult onsets[186].

The behavioural rules are applicable, but they bring fewer benefits.

Drug therapy is an option but must avoid drugs which may be habit forming and/or lead to memory problems.

This insomnia shows weakness in the organization of the Sleep-Wakefulness System.

---

[186] Edinger JD, Manber R, Buysse DJ, Krystal AD, Thase ME, Gehrman P, Fairholme CP, Luther J, Wisniewski S. Are Patients with Childhood Onset of Insomnia and Depression More Difficult to Treat Than Are Those with Adult Onsets of These Disorders? A Report from the TRIAD Study. J Clin Sleep Med. 2017 Feb 15;13(2):205-213. doi: 10.5664/jcsm.6448. PMID: 27784414; PMCID: PMC5263076.

NOTHING I TAKE CAN MAKE ME SLEEP

— I took all possible medications and nothing "makes me" sleep! It started many years ago. My mother was sick, and I took care of her until she died; many nights awake and after she passed away I was really down. The GP told me I should take something, it was lorazepam 1mg; it helped for a while, after some years I should increase the dose... 2mg... and after 2.5 and after 5 ...

The GP said it was too much, it would spoil my memory, and I added alprazolam ... I took both together decreasing lorazepam a little bit and it hold reasonably for 1 year more, and then again no effect. I was depressed for the second time ...

— When was the first depression?

— After my mother's death. The GP said I should consult a psychiatrist; he gave me mirtazapine[187]

— Did you increase your weight?

— Yes, indeed I got some extra pounds, and the depression increased in parallel with the increased size of my clothes. I never went back to my previous weight. But then I took some antidepressants, several I don't remember the names but I took the list. I changed the Psychiatrist 2 or 3 times; I went to 2 Neurologists ... I don't remember the names ... someone gave me something like risperidone[188] and another named ... quetiapine[189]... You see I took already everything and no effects, no results, nothing my nights are a martyrdom ... a eyes wide open nightmare ... I hate my bed so much that I sleep now in the sofa with the TV all night long ... but even so I don't sleep ... I think I will die soon with so many sleepless

---

[187] Remeron
[188] Risperdal
[189] Seroquel

nights ... I am desperate ... no hope ... no will to do what so ever ... during the day I try to sleep and lay down ... but even so I don't sleep. My sleep is gone, it abandoned me, and I am lost ... please give me something that really makes me sleep...
— What are you taking at present?
— 2 lorazepam[190], 2 alprazolam[191], 200g quetiapine altogether at bedtime and venlafaxine[192] 150mg at breakfast

Many randomized controlled trials support the efficacy of approved pharmacological treatments, namely, benzodiazepine (BZD) and non-benzodiazepine (non-BZD), GABA-A modulators, dual orexin receptor antagonists (DORAs), melatonin receptor agonists and histamine antagonists[193].

However, long term use of insomnia medication is not recommended[194].

BZDs, such as lorazepam and alprazolam, are GABA modulators, and as such cause cause sedation, anticonvulsant, anxiolytic, and muscle relaxant effects. They increase brain fast activity, render sleep more superficial and depress breathing amplitude while reducing respiratory reflexes, i.e., they increase the risk of sleep apnea; furthermore, they might facilitate sleep onset, but they induce habituation and dependence, i.e., the tendency to increase the dose and the inability to sleep without them. Daytime aftereffects affect daytime vigilance and increase the risk of accidents and lapses, together with a negative impact upon memory.

---

[190] Lorenin, Ativan or Orvidal
[191] Xanax, Xanax XR
[192] Effexor, Effexor XR and Trevilor
[193] Rosenberg, R.; Citrome, L.; Drake, C.L. Advances in the Treatment of Chronic Insomnia: A Narrative Review of New Nonpharmacologic and Pharmacologic Therapies. Neuropsychiatr. Dis. Treat. 2021, 17, 2549–2566.
[194] Zee PC, Bertisch SM, Morin CM, Pelayo R, Watson NF, Winkelman JW, Krystal AD. Long-Term Use of Insomnia Medications: An Appraisal of the Current Clinical and Scientific Evidence. J Clin Med. 2023 Feb 17;12(4):1629. doi: 10.3390/jcm12041629. PMID: 36836164; PMCID: PMC9959182.

BZDs are not recommended in older adults[194,195] due to the risks of falls, the memory impact and dementia risk[196].

Non-BZDs study results showed dose-dependent sustained improvement in self-reported sleep onset and maintenance in non-elderly and elderly patients. No rebound insomnia was observed, and adverse events were mild and dose-dependent[194].

A controlled study proved that long term use of hypnotics increased significantly the risk of cancer and of premature death and the risk was dose dependent[197]; the cancer risk was not found in other studies[198]

Doxepin, is a GAGA-A modulator and a tricyclic antidepressant, showed a sustained improvement in most clinical endpoints, (sleep maintenance and healthcare professional- and patient-reported ratings on awakening). A favourable risk-to-benefit ratio was sustained over 12 weeks [194]

For sedating antidepressant there is only scant evidence for indicating sedating antidepressants in the treatment of insomnia. Significant but small effects were noted for doxepin and trazodone

[195] Riemann D, Espie CA, Altena E, Arnardottir ES, Baglioni C, Bassetti CLA, Bastien C, Berzina N, Bjorvatn B, Dikeos D, Dolenc Groselj L, Ellis JG, Garcia-Borreguero D, Geoffroy PA, Gjerstad M, Gonçalves M, Hertenstein E, Hoedlmoser K, Hion T, Holzinger B, Janku K, Jansson-Fröjmark M, Järnefelt H, Jernelöv S, Jennum PJ, Khachatryan S, Krone L, Kyle SD, Lancee J, Leger D, Lupusor A, Marques DR, Nissen C, Palagini L, Paunio T, Perogamvros L, Pevernagie D, Schabus M, Shochat T, Szentkiralyi A, Van Someren E, van Straten A, Wichniak A, Verbraecken J, Spiegelhalder K. The European Insomnia Guideline: An update on the diagnosis and treatment of insomnia 2023. J Sleep Res. 2023 Dec;32(6):e14035. doi: 10.1111/jsr.14035. PMID: 38016484.

[196] Tseng, L.Y.; Huang, S.T.; Peng, L.N.; Chen, L.K.; Hsiao, F.Y. Benzodiazepines, z-Hypnotics, and Risk of Dementia: Special Considerations of Half-Lives and Concomitant Use. Neurotherapeutics **2020**, 17, 156–164

[197] Kripke DF, Langer RD, Kline LE. Hypnotics' association with mortality or cancer: a matched cohort study. *BMJ Open.* 2012;**2**:e000850.

[198] Pottegård A, Friis S, Andersen M, Hallas J. Use of benzodiazepines or benzodiazepine related drugs and the risk of cancer: a population-based case-control study. Br J Clin Pharmacol. 2013 May;75(5):1356-64. doi: 10.1111/bcp.12001. PMID: 23043261; PMCID: PMC3635606.

in the short term, up to 4 weeks. Sedating antidepressant should be used in comorbid insomnia and depression[195].

Melatonin agonists like, Ramelteon over the 6 months of treatment, reduced sleep onset (latency to persistent sleep assessed by polysomnography and subjective sleep latency) when compared to placebo with no significant next-morning residual effects, rebound insomnia or withdrawal symptoms[194].

Melatonin: there small to medium effects on sleep-related parameters in elderly patients and patients with insomnia, in short-term studies. Melatonin is manufactured by very different sources and can be purchased through a variety of avenues like supermarkets, internet, chemists and pharmacies, likely resulting in marked variations in pharmacological quality[195].

Herbal remedies/ phytotherapeutics: There is evidence from low-quality original studies of diverse plant cocktails. Therefore herbal/ phytotherapeutic interventions cannot be recommended for either short- or long-term use to treat insomnia[195].

Antihistamines, include Diphenhydramine, doxylamine, hydroxyzine, promethazine. At present, the scientific evidence does not support a recommendation for antihistaminergic drugs in the treatment of insomnia either short or long term[195].

Antipsychotics: the scientific evidence does not recommend the use of antipsychotics (including quetiapine) in the treatment of insomnia without comorbidities, in either the short or long term[195].

The DORA (drug orexin receptor antagonist) include Suvorexant, Lemborexant, Daridorexant

Suvorexant at 30–40 mg was efficacious for subjective measures of sleep onset and maintenance insomnia, and safe over 1 year of nightly treatment[194].

Lemborexant with 5 and 10 mg doses significant benefits were obtained in objective and subjective measures in sleep efficiency and wake after sleep onset compared to a placebo[194].

Daridorexant improved sleep quality measures and daytime functioning in patients with insomnia[194].

Excessive medication prevents sleep, modifies sleep patterns and has important side effects. Furthermore, the high dosages without effect give the patient a hopeless view of his/her situation.

BZD are not recommended in long term treatments (patient is taking lorazepam and alprazolam).

Antidepressants (patient is taking venlafaxine) are recommended in the presence of comorbid depression. They reduce REM sleep, they might reduce sexual drive, increase weight, fatigue or insomnia, provoke dry mouth, dizziness or constipation.

Antipsychotics like quetiapine in the high dosages have several side effects, among which the more common and less serious are chills, cold sweats, confusion, dizziness, faintness, or lightheadedness when getting up suddenly from a lying or sitting position, sleepiness or unusual drowsiness; however serious side effects and signs of toxicity are seizures, decreased urine, dry mouth, increased thirst, mood changes, muscle pain or cramps, nausea or vomiting, numbness or tingling in the hands, feet, or lips and weakness.

Overall, this patient will have a reduction in sleep duration, a reduction in REM and Slow wave sleep, reduced sleep efficiency and frequent awakenings after sleep onset. The sleep EEG will have superimposed abundant fast rhythms, which might coincide with some diffuse increase of theta (slow) activity. A respiratory hypoventilation is possible with increased number of sleep apneas.

Treatment is complex but will imply a change in daily habits, progressive reduction of medication, cognitive behavior therapy and close patient support.

If you suffer from insomnia take care with excessive medication

I AM A MESS

I don't sleep! I simply don't sleep.

Whatever I do, I can't sleep.

I stay up all night. Nights on end without sleeping, so many that I am afraid I won't be able to handle it.

Nobody can handle so many nights without sleeping.

I have tried everything, including strong medication.

An orthopaedic surgeon gave me dormicum and assured me: "this will definitely get you to sleep".

Come again? Nothing, my eyes didn't close once during the night. It even seemed to get worse.

I went to Orthopaedics because of my bones. I've got arthritis and a lack of calcium in my bones.

But prior to that the General Practitioner had given me Xanax and Sedoxil, and they had not worked.

The Psychiatrist first prescribed Sedoxil and another drug I don't remember and then told me: "this will definitely get you to sleep". He gave me some drops. I think that was how it was?!... that was it. I took 10 drops at the beginning and slept for about 3 hours, but after that I did not sleep so well. But I still take them to sleep.

My body just can't take that many more years without sleeping.

Then I have a lot of illnesses. I have high blood pressure, a stomach ulcer... or in the.... How is it called?... that's it, in the duodenum, more reflux, it's a burning sensation that I can't even begin to describe.

Asthma - I have also had asthma and bone spurs in my spine. It seems that my column is a mess. I have chest pain and I'm fat, of course I'm fat. I can't do anything.

The only thing that gives me any pleasure are the morning programmes, those... on... what's his name... it's slipped my tongue

I don't even enjoy watching the soaps, because I am so depressed. Really, really depressed. No wish to do anything, no wish to talk to anybody. I just want to be alone without anybody saying anything to me.

The Psychiatrist doesn't know what to do with me. He has changed my pills to see if it will have any effect, but nothing. Then I have dizzy spells. I went to the ENT specialist and he prescribed Vastarel and Betaserc. But I also went to the Neurologists. I get this shaking in my hands. It's really complicated drinking tea – I spill half in the saucer.

Now my husband says that my mouth twitches in a funny way.

Well I just don't know, I'm a mess. I don't think I can take it any longer without sleeping.

"And what medication are you currently taking?"

"Look Doctor, I've got everything written down here because there are so many different pills, some for my head, some for my bones, and so on. I've got it on this piece of paper (shows a piece of paper listing the considerable number of pills she is taking).

I also have some exams. I did a CT scan on the head and everything. I've got lots of ailments and I've got my blood and urine tests here. I've got high cholesterol. Do you want to see?"

This patient has a lot of complaints:

- *Osteoporosis and osteoarticular pains and problems.*
- *Hypertension. Hypercholesterolemia.*
- *Asthma and chest pain*
- *Gastrointestinal ulcer and gastro-oesophageal reflux problems.*
- *Trembling and possibly tongue dyskinesias.*
- *Vertigos or dizziness.*
- *Depression.*
- *Insomnia.*
- *Polypharmacy.*

This is a common situation in the daily life of a doctor. These patients go from doctor to doctor and at each clinical unit they are prescribed pills which over time may lead to other situations, due to associated side effects.

There is no systematisation of these problems nor a global management of them, and in the current stage one of the main problems is polypharmacy.

Patients are convinced that pills for the head are for the head, those for the stomach are for the stomach, those for the bones for the bones, etc., and that as a result pills do not mix or interact. This is not true, as pills get mixed when absorbed into the stomach or the intestine, into the blood stream and in excretion, that is, into the liver or the kidney.

There is no objective scientific knowledge to explain the interactions of such a large number of medications. Most interactions that are known have to do with pairs of medications.

This patient is of a certain age, and this situation is common in elderly people but can occur in younger individuals around 40 or 50. In the elderly, polypharmacy is even more serious, because the body takes longer to eliminate a lot of drugs and is less effective.

In countries like Portugal the rates of polypharmacy are relatively alarming.

The specific sleep disturbance in this case is linked to several medical illnesses and polypharmacy. It is not a primary problem. A number of the drugs that the patient is taking cause insomnia. Many of the complaints that the patient has cause sleep disturbances.

One of the possible solutions in this case is to gradually reduce the patient's medication, removing non-essential medication, and monitoring the evolution of the complaints.

This patient should be monitored through a joint multidisciplinary approach, involving Internists, Psychiatrists and Neurologists.

Improvement following reduction of medication is normally substantial.

<u>A high medication burden is often more harmful than useful</u>.

I CANNOT SLEEP, BUT I DO SLEEP BETTER AT MY BROTHER'S

I am 75 years old

I have always had an active life. I worked a lot and occupied some very important positions. I never got married, but I was quite successful with women. I dedicated my life to work and a few hobbies. I collect coins and old prints, good restaurants, good wines, and some fun.

But the last few years have been difficult.

I only manage to fall asleep at 5:00 am or 6:00 am morning, when dawn breaks and then I wake up at around 3:00 or 4:00 pm and have a light breakfast. Then I still go down to the office to see what is going on. I have dinner at 10:00 pm in a restaurant near my house and I eat and drink something. I like to drink a fine wine and a good brandy.

I go home and entertain myself watching TV and try and read something and then the cycle starts over again.

Yes, I live alone. As I mentioned, I never got married. I don't have any children, but I have some nephews and nieces that I really love.

What is curious is that when I go back to where I was brought up - I am from the North, and I sleep in my brother's house - I fall asleep peacefully at a decent hour.

In my home I am alone at night. It would be not funny that someone would find me dead in the morning...

Usually, I fell asleep at dawn, the night can be a little bit frightening...

This patient has symptoms of a sleep phase delay syndrome, which onset in old age is rare, together with marked errors in sleep hygiene (a single and late hot meal (the late dinner) with wine and brandy).

With age there is a tendency to fall asleep and wake up earlier, that is, to bring the sleep phase forward (advanced sleep delay syndrome).

In this case the eveningness and the strange fact of sleeping well in the family home immediately suggests a fear of sleeping alone and dying in one's sleep, as referred by the patient at the end.

In this description some aspects must be considered: the sleep resistance, the fear of the dark and the fear of dying in his sleep.

Sleep resistance and fear of sleep associated with panic symptoms (sweating, faster heart rate, shortness of breath, tremor) are called Somnophobia[199]. It occurs in children, adolescents, or adults with intense and threatening nightmares and in Post Traumatic Stress Disorder.

Death anxiety or thanatophobia is a possible cause of insomnia and may be associated with a "loud ego"[200], as the patient also expressed

The fear of dying in one's sleep is not uncommon in elderly individuals, especially if they live alone.

It may also occur in individuals with heart problems and a family history of sudden deaths.

This fear may lead to insomnia or to an inversion in the sleep cycle: you remain awake when you are alone and start sleeping when the day arrives, and people are around.

---

[199] Somniphobia: Understanding the Fear of Sleep (sleepfoundation.org)

[200] Watson, N.F. Insomnia and Death Anxiety: A Theoretical Model with Therapeutic Implications. J. Clin. Med. **2023**, 12, 3250. https://doi.org/10.3390/jcm12093250

Furthermore, errors in sleep hygiene[201] and a disturbed circadian clock, reduction in melatonin production, lower sensitivity to light, lower light exposure, a poor interaction between the circadian and the homeostatic system common in elderly people are other contributing causes[202].

The solutions for these cases are complex and each case must be dealt on individually.

The fear of dying in one's sleep is a possible cause of insomnia or having a late sleep.

---

[201] Irish LA, Kline CE, Gunn HE, Buysse DJ, Hall MH. The role of sleep hygiene in promoting public health: A review of empirical evidence. Sleep Med Rev. 2015 Aug;22:23-36. doi: 10.1016/j.smrv.2014.10.001. Epub 2014 Oct 16. PMID: 25454674; PMCID: PMC4400203.

[202] Duffy JF, Zitting KM, Chinoy ED. Aging and Circadian Rhythms. Sleep Med Clin. 2015 Dec;10(4):423-34. doi: 10.1016/j.jsmc.2015.08.002. Epub 2015 Sep 15. PMID: 26568120; PMCID: PMC4648699.

I USED TO SLEEP WELL, NOT NOW

I don't know what I've got. I've been irritable, tired. I've got headaches, and most of all I can't sleep. I used to sleep well. Even when I had children I continued to sleep well. I have friends of mine who did not sleep at that time, but not me.

I don't have any problems in life, I get on well with my husband, work is fine and the children are just wonderful.

I don't have any reasons not to sleep, and I do not understand what this means. I don't feel ill, I've had blood and urine tests and everything is fine. My thyroid is fine, my GP is very careful and made me do a battery of tests. I did a CT scan and a EEG because of the headaches and everything is normal. I don't have any problems with my spine.

I don't work too much, and leave at 5:00 pm, get the children and then we go home. I make dinner while they do their homework, then my husband arrives and we have dinner.

Then I sort out the kitchen with him and we watch a little TV. Sometimes there are arguments... it's just that he falls asleep immediately and there is no chance to talk. He hasn't fallen asleep and he is already snoring. We argue about that, because he claims he doesn't snore, but he does.

He snores so much, and hasn't the faintest idea, and he has snored for years and years. Before it wasn't a problem, namely when I used to sleep well. He could snore at will, then there was a stage when he would only go to bed after I had fallen asleep. But now that something is not right with me, I can't handle the noise.

In the middle of the night, I go to the living room and sleep on the sofa. He doesn't believe it, says that I am exaggerating, but the other day the neighbours living above us complained. He was very perplexed at that and started thinking that there must be something wrong with him, but he wants me to get sorted first and he says then it will be his turn.

Chronic sleep deprivation of snorers bedpartners, both in terms of hours slept and in terms of the lightness of sleep, has been scientifically proved in these cases.

Wives (and husbands) of snorers have chronic sleep deprivation, because they are daily subject to an intense nocturnal noise.[203]

Bed partners of untreated OSAS patients and patients with heavy snoring are three time more likely to report insomnia, twice more likely to report daytime and health consequences (fatigue, sleepiness, increased weight) and worse quality of life[204].

The disturbance reasons are snoring (69%), apneas (54%), and restlessness (55%)

Partners can positively and negatively influence patients' adoption and use of OSA treatments.

Snoring, as mentioned above, is mainly bad for the snorer, but the person sleeping alongside does not remain free of its effects. In these cases, it is essential to treat the companion.

If you have insomnia, see if your partner snores and convince him to be treated!

---

[203] When Your Partner Snores, No One Sleeps (sleepfoundation.org)
[204] Luyster FS. Impact of Obstructive Sleep Apnea and Its Treatments on Partners: A Literature Review. J Clin Sleep Med. 2017 Mar 15;13(3):467-477. doi: 10.5664/jcsm.6504. PMID: 28095973; PMCID: PMC5337594.

3. STRANGE MOVEMENTS DURING SLEEP

Sleep-related movement disorders of the adult include restless legs syndrome (RLS; Willis-Ekbom disease), periodic limb movement disorder, sleep-related bruxism, sleep-related leg cramps, and, rhythmic movement disorder in children and presently restless sleep syndrome (see D,4).

They are characterized by simple repetitive movements, like a quick jerk, a twitch, sudden turn, teeth clenching, a rhythmic movement, which interfere with sleep.

Movements fragment or interrupt sleep inducing insomnia complaints and daytime consequences, such as fatigue, depression, headaches, concentration problems, etc. The bedpartners may not notice small amplitude movements or may be extremely distressed with the movement's agitation.

I CANNOT STAND MY LEGS

My headaches are unbearable. They start in the morning and get worse throughout the day. I'm worse.

But how long has it been? Maybe 2 years ago. Before, they were spaced out, but now they are constant.

Do I have a brain tumor? I've already done CT scans, but maybe I should do an MRI.

I am always tired. I don't feel like doing anything.

The other day I slapped Richard. He was irritating me... he knows how to do it ... but I was annoyed, slapping is not OK.

I don't know what to do anymore. I don't feel like doing anything. I'm tired, I don't feel like talking to anyone. If only I could sleep and be well!

It takes me hours to fall asleep, and I can only sleep at dawn, but then, when I'm finally sleeping well, I have to get up; so..., in the morning I'm still more tired than when I went to bed.

What a bummer. I must teach and put up with all the demands.

If I could sleep and be well. Falling asleep is an ordeal, I must put my legs out of bed to cool them down. The students are unbearable. Putting up with them, tired and with headaches is an ordeal. Legs are scalding. I'm going to get up and walk around a little to see if it goes away. There is nothing to eat in the fridge. What a bummer! It's better to go back to bed.

Restless legs syndrome (RLS) is very common[205,206,207], but often unrecognized, both by patients and medical doctors. This patient only refers RLS symptoms at the end of her complaint report. Active questioning to specify the symptoms is required.

RLS has a high prevalence rate of around 5 to 15% of the population, having 1.5 to 2.7% a significant severity, with symptoms occurring 2 or more times per week with moderate distress[205]. Usually it presents in middle-aged patients, around 40-50 years of age.

There is a family history, involving several family members, given the high penetrance of certain genes (Polymorphisms in genes including BTBD9 and MEIS1)[206]. In family cases, the onset age is earlier, in childhood or adolescence.

In non-familiar cases it can be linked to anaemia or low iron and ferritin levels, renal insufficiency, polyneuropathies (that is, illnesses of the peripheral nerves), renal insufficiency, diabetes, venous insufficiency, fibromyalgia, amyloidosis, lumbosacral radiculopathy, celiac disease, folate or magnesium deficiency, and pregnancy[206]. Some medications may cause or aggravate RLS (neuroleptics, some antidepressants, lithium and beta-blockers)[206].

Patients with restless legs syndrome have a restlessness in the legs, which presents when falling asleep or at the end of the day or in period of wakeful rest.

Sensations of pain, burning, tickling or just an inexplicable feeling, an urge to move and relieve with movement are typical.

---

[205] Silber MH, Buchfuhrer MJ, Earley CJ, Koo BB, Manconi M, Winkelman JW; Scientific and Medical Advisory Board of the Restless Legs Syndrome Foundation. The Management of Restless Legs Syndrome: An Updated Algorithm. Mayo Clin Proc. 2021 Jul;96(7):1921-1937. doi: 10.1016/j.mayocp.2020.12.026. PMID: 34218864.

[206] Mansur A, Castillo PR, Rocha Cabrero F, et al. Restless Legs Syndrome. [Updated 2023 Feb 27]. In: StatPearls [Internet]. Treasure Island (FL): StatPearls Publishing; 2024 Jan-. Available from: https://www.ncbi.nlm.nih.gov/books/NBK430878/

[207] Home - Restless Legs Syndrome Foundation (rls.org)

The symptoms improve with moving or walking, and sometimes the patient suddenly gets out of bed and, without any apparent reason, starts walking (akathisia). The unpleasant feelings may be strong enough to require other strategies: legs out of the bed or immersed in cold water or ice, massaging, stretching, etc.

Sleep initiation becomes difficult, and the patient only manages to fall asleep at dawn. When they wake up, they are often tired with headaches. Sleep deprivation gives rise to depression, irritability memory deficits and suicidal risk. In serious cases the impact upon quality of life may be devastating.

Typical difficulties include keeping your legs from moving at the cinema or during evening concerts or long trips.

RLS may be linked to periodic limb movement disorder (PLMD), that is, involuntary leg movements during the night, from one minute to the next, for example, sometimes leading to a micro-awakening.

The association of restless legs with periodic limb movements makes sleep disturbance even more pronounced.

The physiopathology of restless legs is still not well understood. There is a central dysfunction of the dopaminergic system (the putamen and caudate nucleus[208]), with perturbations in central and motor integration, that is, a sensory perturbation (a weird sensation or dysesthesia) transformed into a motor action (an involuntary or irresistible movement); furthermore, there are also errors in the brain's metabolism of iron and iron homeostatic mechanisms; increased cerebral glutamate and decreased adenosine are likely to intervene[205]. Despite these alterations,

---

[208] The putamen and caudate form part of the Basal Ganglia, cerebral structures located at the base of the forebrain, which participate in the regulation of movement and which are altered, for example, in Parkinson's disease. Despite Parkinson's patients having a greater frequency of PLMD, there is no relationship between Restless Leg Syndrome and Parkinson's.

conventional brain imaging tests such as a CT or MRI scan give normal results.

There is specific treatment for RLS.

General measures: Alcohol, tobacco and coffee should be avoided.

Regular exercise significantly improves the symptoms. Daily exercise, namely walking, practised at daytime, is highly recommended since it attenuates the symptoms.

Current pharmacological treatment uses as first line alpha2-delta calcium channels ligands (pregabalin and gabapentin)[205].

Dopaminergic drugs (mostly ropinirole, pramipexole, and rotigotine) are second choice; they are also used in the treatment of Parkinson's Disease, but in RLS they are taken in lower doses and usually before going to bed. The risk of augmentation[209], i.e., increased symptoms severity with increased medication dosage, may occur in rare cases.

Dipyridamole, a blocker of the adenosine reuptake transporters, has a therapeutic effect.

Low dose opioid therapy is recommended in refractory RLS[205].

Treatment of any cause that may be present (anaemia, polyneuropathy, etc.). Serum iron and ferritin must be measured in all cases. In case ferritin is below 75mg/l consider oral therapy with Vit C; consider intravenous therapy in more serious cases[205].

---

[209] Garcia-Borreguero D, Silber MH, Winkelman JW, Högl B, Bainbridge J, Buchfuhrer M, Hadjigeorgiou G, Inoue Y, Manconi M, Oertel W, Ondo W, Winkelmann J, Allen RP. Guidelines for the first-line treatment of restless legs syndrome/Willis-Ekbom disease, prevention and treatment of dopaminergic augmentation: a combined task force of the IRLSSG, EURLSSG, and the RLS-foundation. Sleep Med. 2016 May;21:1-11. doi: 10.1016/j.sleep.2016.01.017. Epub 2016 Feb 23. PMID: 27448465.

In patients with anaemia or low ferritin, iron therapy is very effective and should be considered as the first option[210].

In treatment it is important to understand the evolution and the seriousness of the overall condition, since both vary from patient to patient. In cases where there is a persistent evolution, treatment should be daily, but many cases have spurts in the evolution due to somewhat inexplicable and unpredictable reasons, and at those times treatment should be carried out or higher doses of medication taken.

RLS a frequent complaint, frequently unrecognised

---

[210] Allen RP, Picchietti DL, Auerbach M, Cho YW, Connor JR, Earley CJ, Garcia-Borreguero D, Kotagal S, Manconi M, Ondo W, Ulfberg J, Winkelman JW; International Restless Legs Syndrome Study Group (IRLSSG). Evidence-based and consensus clinical practice guidelines for the iron treatment of restless legs syndrome/Willis-Ekbom disease in adults and children: an IRLSSG task force report. Sleep Med. 2018 Jan;41:27-44. doi: 10.1016/j.sleep.2017.11.1126. Epub 2017 Nov 24. PMID: 29425576.

MY WIFE SAYS I SEEM LIKE A HORSE

Well, I've come here because my wife says that I seem like a horse, and she can't sleep with me.

To be honest, I don't feel anything is wrong with me. I have a busy professional life, and I don't have any serious problems.

I'm worried about the fact I'm disturbing my wife, and lately I have been sleeping in the other room.

She says that I don't snore, and I don't stop breathing.

I don't have sleepiness or memory problems.

Well, may be lately I have been remembering more of my dreams, but I wake up in a good mood... sometimes I have a light headache which goes away as soon as I get up.

I am not excessively sleepy, and I never fall asleep unless I wish to, or when I am not in bed."

"You are going to have to do a polysomnography with video."

....

"I must tell you that your wife is right. You are making very strong movements with your body, which are mainly affecting your legs and, as a result, it reminds a horse's kicking. These are periodic limb movements for which there is a specific treatment."

This example describes a case of Periodic Limb Movement Disorder (PLMD) [211,212]***.***

---

[211] Joseph V, Nagalli S. Periodic Limb Movement Disorder. [Updated 2023 Feb 14]. In: StatPearls [Internet]. Treasure Island (FL): StatPearls Publishing; 2024 Jan-. Available from: https://www.ncbi.nlm.nih.gov/books/NBK560727/

[212] O'Regan D, Anderson KN. Restless legs syndrome and periodic limb movements of sleep. Br J Hosp Med (Lond). 2020 Jan 2;81(1):1-8. doi: 10.12968/hmed.2019.0319. Epub 2020 Jan 28. PMID: 32003620.

PLMDs are a frequent sleep pathology. Prevalence estimates range from 4 to 11%, with lower values in African Americans in comparison with Caucasian Americans.

PLMDs generally occur associated with Restless Legs Syndrome, narcolepsy, sleep apnoeas[213], ADHD, RBD (REM Behaviour Disorder), uraemia and spinal tumour[211]. In a specific number of patients, not presenting with any other pathology, this constitutes the dominant condition, primary PLMD.

It consists of short, periodic and stereotyped movements at regular intervals of approximately 1 minute, which affect the lower limbs, such as flexing the foot, the leg and the thigh. It can affect one or both legs and the arms as well. They are often not very extensive and as such, contrary to this case history, they can go unnoticed both by patients and by those sleeping with them. Partner who shares the bed may notice leg stretching or can complain of being kicked.

They are involuntary movements.

PLMDs should be suspected when there are morning complaints of morning fatigue or headaches or when the person states that they wake up more tired than when they went to bed.

The risk factors are low iron and low ferritin, low magnesium, medications like dopamine blockers, antidepressants (TCAs and SSRIs), older age, male gender, obesity, diabetes, stress, caffein consumption, shift work and some genes[211] and the use of CPAP in sleep apnea patients without PLMS at baseline[212].

Treatment is carried is similar rules to those of Restless Legs Syndrome; some other medications are advised: clonazepam, melatonin, sodium valproate and selegiline. Alcohol and coffee should be avoided. Exercise is beneficial.

<u>It is not just snoring that can disturb your partner. Being kicked can do it as well.</u>

213

SHE GRINDS HER TEETH

I have always ground my teeth. That is, my mother says that as a child I always made a lot of noise.

It goes through certain phases of life. When I am tense it's worse. I end up waking up with my face aching.

It seems that I have been grinding my teeth throughout the night, sometimes at the beginning and at other times at the end, and others during the night. I know this because that is what they tell me, as I don't wake up.

In fact, I sleep well, fall asleep quickly and generally don't wake up. Sometimes I wake up with somewhat of a heavy head ... it doesn't hurt; other times I feel a bit of pain in my face muscles in the morning, as I've already said.

I don't have any other complaints.

Well ... my teeth are a bit ruined, but I've never broken any of them. My dentist is always complaining.

I must admit I've never paid much attention to it, but I've now got married and my husband can't stand the noise. He says that I'm preventing him from sleeping and that the noise is unpleasant.

So that's why I've come here, to see if you can help me.

The patient has a condition which is known as bruxism[214], named after the rather creepy noise made when grinding one's teeth ("the witch's noise"). It involves both rhythmic contractions of the masseter muscles, accompanied by teeth grinding and mandible

---

[214] Lal SJ, Sankari A, Weber, DDS KK. Bruxism Management. [Updated 2024 May 1]. In: StatPearls [Internet]. Treasure Island (FL): StatPearls Publishing; 2024 Jan-. Available from: https://www.ncbi.nlm.nih.gov/books/NBK482466/

thrusting (phasic bruxism) or tonic persistent contractions of the masseter muscles (tonic bruxism).

Sleep bruxism is most common in children, affecting 15% to 40% of children and 8% to 10% of adults[214].

Familiar prevalence: 20% to 50% of patients report at least 1 family member with bruxism. A genome-wide association study reveals a significant correlation between the rs10193179 variant of the Myosin IIIB gene (MYO3B) and sleep bruxism[214].

This condition may be related to bad dental occlusion and with other sleep disorders, but may also occur without any apparent cause.

Obstructive sleep apnea, restless leg syndrome, periodic limb movement, sleep-related gastroesophageal reflux disease, REM behavior disorder, and sleep-related epilepsy are associated with sleep bruxism[214].

Medications and drugs may increase bruxism: amphetamines, antipsychotics, antidepressants, cocaine and 3,4-methylenedioxymethamphetamine[214].

Patients sometimes complain of pain in the masticatory muscles in the morning, and the force may be so strong that it can break a tooth. The teeth appear fractured, as if cut in the middle, and it is essential to protect them with a dental guard.

Bruxism is an involuntary movement and, while it can be accentuated during periods of psychological tension, it is not caused by being nervous, although there is the idea of there being personality patterns associated with it, which are more tense and more restrained, involving difficulty in expressing emotions.

It may temporarily occur in children, which does not require specific treatment, except to protect the teeth, so as not to lead to any deterioration in the enamel.

Dental treatments, especially stabilization splints, represent a safe and relatively effective management approach to reduce EMG- based SB frequency and intensity. Dental treatments are more effective than pharmacological or behavioural treatment.

Grinding your teeth will ruin them.

4. Pain and Sleep

Pain and Sleep have mutual negative influences

Nocturnal pain impacts negatively upon sleep and a disturbed sleep impacts upon daily pain.

Sleep disturbance predicts daily pain in the subsequent day, but the opposite does not hold, ie, the intensity of pain does not predict subsequent sleep quality.

Musculoskeletal pain particularly affects sleep.

Headaches also since they can wake up patients during the night and disturb sleep. Headaches may be a cause of bad sleep, and whenever sleep problems and headache overlap the prognosis of headache treatment is poorer.

MY HEAD AND MY SLEEP ARE KILLING ME

The headaches are unbearable. They start in the morning and get worse throughout the day. I've got worse. But for how long?

May be 2 years. Previously they were spaced out but now they are constant.

Could I have a tumour!?

I've already had a brain CT scan but perhaps I need to do an MRI scan.

I am tired. I don't feel like doing anything. The other day I slapped Richard. He was asking for it, but I've been a bit irritable lately.

I don't know what to do. I don't feel like doing anything. I'm tired and I don't feel like talking to anyone.

If I could just manage to sleep and be OK!

It takes hours for me to fall asleep and I only manage to drop off at dawn, but then, when I am finally sleeping well, I must get up. That is why I am more tired in the morning than when I went to bed.

As I don't sleep I eat something to calm down... cookies, chocolate...

What a drag! I must give my classes! Putting up with students and all their demands! If I could just manage to sleep and feel OK!

Falling asleep is a torture. I must put my legs outside the bed to cool them down.

The students are unbearable. Putting up with them when tired and with a headache is a torture.

My legs are scalding. I'm going to get up and walk a little and see if that makes a difference.

There's nothing to eat in the fridge. Cookies are over! What a drag! I might as well go back to bed.

This patient has several complaints: frequent and severe headaches starting upon waking, which are called morning headaches; irritability and depressive symptoms; insomnia; possible restless legs; nocturnal eating.

These different manifestations interact with each other.

Morning headaches usually reflect a sleep disturbance, and this case has several. The prevalence of morning headaches in European countries in 8% and they were associated anxiety and depressive symptoms, insomnia, sleep-related breathing disorders, hypertension, use of psychotropic medication and heavy alcohol consumption[215]. Morning headaches are the most frequent headache type in Obstructive Sleep Apnea[216]. In Austria morning headaches were associated with "regular use of sleep medication, disturbed sleep, sleep maintenance, tossing and turning around during night and a decreased feeling of refreshment in the morning"[217].

Patients with restless legs have a higher probability of having headaches and patients with headaches associated with a sleep disorder have worse prognosis and more severe headaches. Restless legs and insomnia are often associated due to the increased sleep latency provoked by restless legs and the possible

[215] Ohayon MM. Prevalence and risk factors of morning headaches in the general population. Arch Intern Med 2004; 164:97–102.

[216] Błaszczyk B, Martynowicz H, Więckiewicz M, Straburzyński M, Antolak M, Budrewicz S, Staszkiewicz M, Kopszak A, Waliszewska-Prosół M. Prevalence of headaches and their relationship with obstructive sleep apnea (OSA) - Systematic review and meta-analysis. Sleep Med Rev. 2024 Feb;73:101889. doi: 10.1016/j.smrv.2023.101889. Epub 2023 Dec 1. PMID: 38056382.

[217] Seidel S, Klösch G, Moser D, Weber M, Anderer P, Wöber C, Zeitlhofer J. Morning headaches, daytime functioning and sleep problems--a population-based controlled study. Wien Klin Wochenschr. 2010 Oct;122(19-20):579-83. doi: 10.1007/s00508-010-1464-4. Epub 2010 Sep 30. PMID: 20872079.

association with periodic limb movements of sleep[218], which often provoke maintenance insomnia. In adults and in children morning headaches are significantly associated with periodic limb movements of sleep[219].

Finally nocturnal eating syndromes are also often associated with periodic movements of sleep, as in this patient.

All these disturbances have consequences upon patient humour; irritability and depression are common.

In synthesis sleep disorders are somewhat ubiquitarian, i.e., they can coexist together and add up their effects, with a reinforcement of negative consequences (in this case headache and depression) and increased severity. Treatment must be based in an adequate and tailored strategy.

Sleep disturbances and headaches go often together

---

[218] Joseph V, Nagalli S. Periodic Limb Movement Disorder. [Updated 2023 Feb 14]. In: StatPearls [Internet]. Treasure Island (FL): StatPearls Publishing; 2024 Jan-. Available from: https://www.ncbi.nlm.nih.gov/books/NBK560727/

[219] Delrosso LM, Lockhart C, Wrede JE, Chen ML, Samson M, Reed J, Martin-Washo S, Arp M, Ferri R. Comorbidities in children with elevated periodic limb movement index during sleep. Sleep. 2020 Feb 13;43(2):zsz221. doi: 10.1093/sleep/zsz221. PMID: 31555831.

I DON'T KNOW WHAT COMES FIRST: THE PAIN OR THE INSOMNIA

I have Rheumatoid Arthritis, for more than a decade. I am currently doing the required treatments but nowadays things are not going well.

I am used to pain, and I learned to live with it. But at present I have problems in my work. They treat me well and they have consideration for my work.

The problem is that I feel I am far behind the intended achievements.

I work in social rehabilitation of immigrants. The work per se is not easy, and nowadays with the budget cuts we cannot do much. So, all the plans developed in the last years are kept at the drawer due to the lack of money.

This is very distressing, since I know that our actions would have been useful and would allow sparing of costs in other fields, such as social security and health. It is a pity somehow, but I should be used to the inconsistencies of public administration, since I work in it for several decades, almost 3 at present.

Furthermore, I have problems with my family. I live alone, since I left my parents' house long time ago, but as they are becoming older, they worry that I am not married having nobody to take care of me, and that I don't take care of them, now they start having some health problems.

I must say that my disease is, per itself a big burden for me, which I had to handle the best I could.

But now everything becomes difficult, more difficult.

I don't sleep. The pain becomes unbearable at night. My fingers are tight, and the hands stiff, as if something is blocking the movements with a special strength. Erratic and sharp like pains travel across my limbs. I remain thinking in all my problems trying to find a solution. My thoughts are grey and repetitive. With the same sentences circling in my head again, and again. It is always the same thing: my parents, my work, the immigrants. Moving and turning in bed is difficult. I have no position for my arms or legs, since, whatever I do they hurt.

I cannot take more analgesics, since the stomach is complaining.

Therefore, I don't know whether it is the pain that prevents my sleep, or my sleep that enhances the pain.

The relationship between sleep and pain has been known for years. Pain and Sleep disturbances are considered co-morbid disorders since both are commonly reported problems in clinical practice, emerge associated in epidemiologic studies and cause considerable social and family problems, as well as socio-economic impact and costs.

Chronic pain patients report more daytime symptoms like fatigue, tiredness or sleepiness, depression and insomnia. The quality of sleep has consequences upon pain intensity the next day: worse sleep more intense will be the pain. Furthermore, chronic sleep deprivation is a risk factor for chronic pain.

The neural mechanisms underlying such close relationship are quite complex and multifactorial: 1) inadequate sleep deteriorates functioning of the opioid antinociceptive system; 2) disturbances the serotonergic system, which is involved in both pain and sleep-wake control, may mediate the hyperalgesia of deficient sleep; 3) sleep deficiency enhances pain through increased adenosine activity; 4) Together with adenosine, Nitric Oxide(NO) is an important player in the homeostatic regulation and might be an important pain activator in sleep deprivation; 5) furthermore the orexinergic system is involved in pain transmission and modulation; 6) insomnia symptoms, mild increases in basal cortisol levels and a hyper-reactivity of the HPA (Hypothalamus-pituitary-adrenal) axis to stressors; such hyper-reactivity has been found to mediate the relationship between deficient sleep and higher pain sensitivity; 7) low-grade inflammation, occurring in chronic sleep deprivation, may constitute a mechanism that links short or disturbed sleep to chronic pain.

Altogether, these complex interactions between sleep and pain, besides deserving more studies, show the strength of their mutual interactions[220].

In Rheumatoid Arthritis understanding these interactions is critical for patients' improvement[221].

<u>Bad sleep, worse pain!</u>

---

[220] Haack M, Simpson N, Sethna N, Kaur S, Mullington J. Sleep deficiency and chronic pain: potential underlying mechanisms and clinical implications. Neuropsychopharmacology. 2020 Jan;45(1):205-216. doi: 10.1038/s41386-019-0439-z. Epub 2019 Jun 17. PMID: 31207606; PMCID: PMC6879497.

[221] Irwin MR, Straub RH, Smith MT. Heat of the night: sleep disturbance activates inflammatory mechanisms and induces pain in rheumatoid arthritis. Nat Rev Rheumatol. 2023 Sep;19(9):545-559. doi: 10.1038/s41584-023-00997-3. Epub 2023 Jul 24. PMID: 37488298.

A BOMB IS EXPLODING IN MY HEAD

Francis: You have no idea what has been happening to me recently. I don't know how to explain it well. It isn't exactly a pain, but more like a bomb has gone off in my head. It's a weird noise, which happens when I am falling asleep and of course I wake up immediately. Nobody could sleep with that and then I am afraid of falling asleep in case it happens again. It's a bomb, you see, and it blows up in my head. Nobody has told me what I have, but I have checked on the Internet and I think I know what it is.

John: I would also like to know what that is, as nobody has managed to explain it to me. I never get headaches, except for one situation when, after waking, I huddle up again trying to go back to sleep. It has nothing to do with sleep duration, because there are days in which I sleep for hours on and it happens, and other days I just sleep a few hours and it also happens. It has nothing to do with drinking alcohol, because it happens when I haven't drunk. It has nothing to do with the hour I wake up because it can happen both when I wake up early as well as when I wake up late. Nobody knows what it is, but it is also true that it does not happen very often, and mainly when I cover my head and snuggle down to get a bit more sleep.

In the case of Francis, he has explosion head syndrome[222]. This is a rare condition that consists of the sensation that there is a bomb going off in your head, without pain, and which occurs upon falling asleep or less frequently upon awakening. It is more frequent in elderly persons but can occur in young people. Sometimes it is associated with sleep paralysis, sleep jerks, flashes or fear. It is important to find triggers and to reassure the patient, explaining that there is no harm. Patients find strategies to prevent this

---

[222] Khan I, Slowik JM. Exploding Head Syndrome. [Updated 2022 Dec 12]. In: StatPearls [Internet]. Treasure Island (FL): StatPearls Publishing; 2024 Jan-. Available from: https://www.ncbi.nlm.nih.gov/books/NBK560817/

situation. Painkillers, due to the way they work, are useless. Other possible medications include amitriptyline, clomipramine, topiramate, duloxetine and nifedipine; the rarity of the condition does not allow precise recommendations.

John's situation is a very rare condition, whose aetiology is unknown, and which is known as "Turtle Headache"[223], that is it occurs when, just as with turtles, you shrink your neck to fall back asleep. The criteria for diagnosis are the occurrence on at least 10 days a month for greater than 3 months and last for 15 minutes up to 4 hours after waking. Patient should try not to pull their blankets over their head while in bed, keeping a good sleep hygiene and practising exercise.

If you feel an explosion in your head at sleep onset, don't think you are going mad. Seak advice and treatment

---

[223] Patel P, Prabhu A, Tadi P. Turtle Headache. [Updated 2023 Jul 3]. In: StatPearls [Internet]. Treasure Island (FL): StatPearls Publishing; 2024 Jan-. Available from: https://www.ncbi.nlm.nih.gov/books/NBK545272/

AT 3AM I WAKE UP WITH A HEADACHE

"I have a lot of complaints and, to tell you the truth, I'm desperate because there does not seem to be any solution for this.

They say that I've got sleep apnoea, and I have been operated on twice, and everything is just the same. I wake up at night with a headache, I get up and I tend to go to the living room and wait for it to pass. I have taken everything you can possibly take for the pain: Paracetamol[224], Aspirin, Sumatriptan[225] and lately I've been taking Metamizole[226]. The pain doesn't go away and I'm afraid, because I know that I woke up because I wasn't breathing and I'm afraid of dying.

It's just that longevity runs in my family: my dad died when he was 98 (he was great!), my grandfather when he was 89, and my mother when she was 94... and... I want to live a few more years. I'm 61. I work out every day. I don't have high blood pressure, my cholesterol is good, I'm not fat and I don't smoke or drink alcoholic beverages... you see, everything is fine and I am very careful with myself... the fact that I could die in my sleep from an apnoea is getting to me.

And it is like this every night - if only it could be once in a while - but no, it is systematic — at 3:00 am there I am out of bed not sleeping, taking pills because of the headache. I won't get back to sleep or then I'll fall asleep some 2 hours later, but I wake up early... I put the youngest child in school, because she starts at half past eight.

---

[224] The other generic name is acetaminophen. The brand names are Aceta; Aspirin-Free Pain Relief; Aspirin-Free Anacin Maximum Strength; Dapacin; Fem-Etts; Genapap; Genapap Extra Strength; Genebs; Genebs Extra Strength; Mapap Regular Strength; Mapap Extra Strength; Maranox; MedaCap; MedaTab; Panadol; Tapanol Regular Strength; Tapanol Extra Strength; Tylenol Caplets; Tylenol Tablets 325 mg; Tylenol Regular Strength; Tylenol Extra Strength.
[225] Imigran, Imitrex
[226] Algozone, Algocalmin, Algopyrin, Analgin, Dipyrone, Novalgin, Neo-Melubrina and Optalgin.

I am ready to have a 3rd operation to stop the apnoeas; the CPAP machine is so discomforting. I've tried several times, but I can't really stand it. I do tell myself that it protects me, that I can breathe well and stop having apnoeas, but despite all the recommendations (I have had very good doctors who have been most attentive), what is certain is that either I end up not being able to fall asleep because that thing is suffocating me, or, if I fall asleep, I wake up after a couple of hours and take the mask off because I can't stand it any longer. But the greatest problem is that, despite that, in the early morning… and this is mathematically precise… three hours after falling asleep, I wake up again because I have stopped breathing, and I've got a headache.

As this will be the 3rd operation, I'd like to know what you think. I've got my tests here which show the apnoeas and, in fact, after the 1st operation the apnoeas got better, as you can see in the sleep tests. In the 2nd operation there was also a small improvement so perhaps with the 3rd it will be "third time lucky" and everything will be alright. I have everything booked or agreed upon. I've done 4 sleep tests in various places and everybody has said the same: I have apnoeas and I should use the CPAP or be operated upon.

I am sorry that I have gone on like this and told you everything one thing after another, it's just that I'm "professional" at this and I know what I need to tell you."

…

"And the headache?"

"It's of the kind where it's a dull pain, a thick head, and I don't have anything, I mean I don't vomit and I'm not in agony, my eyes don't water and my nose doesn't run… it's a dull pain all over my head, but it's a mathematical pain, which comes on at certain times. "

…

"?! I'm not dreaming anything up. They tell me that I have the pain because I stopped breathing."

...

"?! No, I'm not suffocating, and my heart isn't beating, and I'm not sweating... I get a little anxious and I'm a little under the weather because of all of this and because, put simply, it just does not go away and I've already done everything that I can and know of, and what they told me to do. "

"You do not have daytime sleepiness. The sleep tests we have performed only have cardiorespiratory channels. The apnoea indexes in your polysomnography's are all below 7/hour; the snoring index is also relatively low; you do not have significant oxygen desaturations neither hypoxemias. The heart rate evolution through the night is normal. It is unlikely that your headaches are related to sleep apnoeas and they you have the danger of dying in your sleep."

Headaches which occur in individuals in the middle of the night at a more advanced age, typically 2 to 3 hours after falling asleep, without any other symptoms such as being in agony, vomiting, eyes watering, etc., which occur frequently, and lead to the patient waking up for a relatively prolonged period, over 15 minutes, are called hypnic headaches[227].

It is a relatively rare condition which affects both sexes, and which is particularly bothersome for the patient, due to its systematic awakenings.

It is not linked to any intracranial neurological pathology. Sometimes the headaches appear in patients with pain medication abuse. No association with nocturnal oxygen desaturations has

---

[227] Al Khalili Y, Chopra P. Hypnic Headache. [Updated 2023 Apr 10]. In: StatPearls [Internet]. Treasure Island (FL): StatPearls Publishing; 2024 Jan-. Available from: https://www.ncbi.nlm.nih.gov/books/NBK557598/

been proved, or any specific relationships with REM and non REM sleep stages.

Treatment can be tried with caffeine before going to bed, as well as melatonin, indomethacin[228] or lithium[229].

Hypnic headaches are one of the sleep-related headaches.

---

[228] Indocin, Indocid
[229] Eskalith, Lithobid.

MY HEADACHES ARE TERRIBLE

I get so many headaches! I always have a headache, almost daily. It has almost become my natural state. It's been like this for several years, since I was 14 or 15. So it's been 15 years of pain.

I wake up with a headache.

It is as if my head were weighed down, being squeezed by something.

I have difficulty in working and focusing due to the pain.

No, I do not feel anything else, and it does not get worse when I have my periods or at the weekend. Well, noise has an effect.

I work in a TV station. I have a high ranked position, full of responsibility and everybody wants everything for yesterday. It is a good job, but it is always very busy. There is indeed a lot of stress. The deadlines are terrible.

Eating? Meals? Well, more or less. I eat a sandwich and have a coffee when I get to work. Lunch is on the go whenever I can. I do not have anything at teatime and have dinner late.

Sleeping? Well, I sleep badly. I wake up, worrying about work, 1 or 2 times a night. I lie there thinking. Now and then it is hard to fall asleep. I sleep 4 or 5 hours.

Working out? I just don't have time.

Hobbies or interests? I don't have time.

I am just tired. I have started having problems with my memory. I read things and can't recall them. I have already had some problems at work — inexplicable memory lapses.

My headaches worry me. I did a CT scan, and everything was normal. My tests are normal. I don't like taking pills. I don't know what to do.

When I was young, I always did a lot of activities, and I was always on the go. It's like that at home – everybody with lots to do, without stopping. Everybody works hard, but there are no problems or family health issues.

And as I said, when I was young I did so much. I went to school; I attended language classes, played basketball semi-professionally and did some tutoring to younger kids to earn some money.

I had headaches even then. I remember my mother taking me to the doctor and doing some tests on my head which were normal, as far as I can remember. I have been taking pain killers since then and now I regularly take paracetamol or aspirin, or a new one which they have been advertising for headaches ... I don't remember the name.

But when I was young, I had good marks and slept well. I used to go to bed and fall asleep at once, maybe for 6 or 7 hours, when I was at secondary school. At college I slept even less and sometimes did an all-nighter. Sometimes I was sleepy during the day, but coffee and Coca-Cola helped.

I drink several coca-colas each day and if I do not drink any I get even more headaches.

This patient has headaches which are called tension-type headaches[230].

Tension-type headaches result from a persistently maintained contraction of the head muscles. They generally begin at the end of the afternoon or day, but when there has been sleep deprivation, they can start in the morning. Chronic and daily tension-type headaches cause suffering and incapacity, but neurological examinations generally reveal nothing abnormal.

[230] Shah N, Hameed S. Muscle Contraction Tension Headache. [Updated 2023 Jul 16]. In: StatPearls [Internet]. Treasure Island (FL): StatPearls Publishing; 2024 Jan-. Available from: https://www.ncbi.nlm.nih.gov/books/NBK562274/

Tension-type headaches which occur in the morning may be the result of a busy life involving stress, irregular meals, lack of sleep, a worried attitude towards problems, and lack of exercise.

The stress, excessive activities and lack of sleep stem from youth/ adolescence. There is chronic long-term sleep deprivation which is compensated for by coffees and coca-colas, rich in caffeine. The caffeine, besides being a stimulant, is also a sleep inhibitor, and has a certain type of effect in enabling analgesics; therefore, taking analgesics and stimulants together is very common. Deprivation of caffeine, in turn, can lead to headaches, so-called rebound headaches.

Despite the chronic nature of the condition, this patient may be fine with certain small changes in her daily life, behaviour alterations and adjustments in her expectations.

If you have headaches every day look at your daily activities and at your sleep.

HEADACHES ARE MY ALARMCLOCK

— Almost every day I wake up around 6 am with pain and tears in my left eye and a wet nostril. I already know what it is, I have a chronic cluster headache, which happily goes off with Oxygen. I was observed by a Headache specialist, made the required tests and so far, I am used to it. However recently my sleep changed: I wake several times at night and upon wake up tired, my wife tells me I snore. I feel something different is occurring.

— In effect there is an association between Cluster Headache and Sleep Apnoea. But did you have high blood pressure, cholesterol, cardiac problems, heartburn, or any other medical disorder? If not, it is better to check sleep with polysomnography

Some days latter

— Well, you have indeed Sleep Apnoea and it is severe enough to recommend PAP therapy

— OK let's try it and see what happens to the Cluster Headache

Some days latter

— Good morning, Doctor! Things are a little better. I sleep more continuously, I don't snore, the CPAP is boring, but I manage to use it. The headaches remain but they occur latter, around lunch time; at that time is more convenient to use the Oxygen therapy.

— Well then. Three good effects: 1) You sleep better; 2) You are reasonably adapted to the CPAP and have no apnoeas, and 3) Something changed your headache clock, but headaches persist... Thinking it over since you already tried triptans, verapamil, valproic acid and melatonin with no results, I would suggest prednisone, starting with a higher dose for five days and decreasing progressively over time.

Two months latter

— Hello Doctor. I am ok. No headaches and no snoring for 2 months. It is fantastic!

Cluster Headaches[231] **are considered the most severe headaches. The intensity can be so severe that patients to hit the walls with their head or have strange and unusual agitation. These behaviours may induce confusion with psychiatric diagnosis.**

However, in these patients the pain is clear: it unilaterally, over the eye and the forehead; it is a excruciating short lasting pain (up to 180 min), associated with _ipsilateral_ **lacrimation, conjunctival injection, nasal congestion or rhinorrhoea, forehead sweating.**

The temporal occurrence is characteristic: every day at the same hour, mostly during the night, in clusters that can have 1- or 2-months duration and recur every two or three years with identical pattern.

This patient had however a chronic form, almost every day without remissions.

Potential triggers are Alcohol, Smoking, Watching television, Hot weather, Stress, Use of nitroglycerine, Sexual activity, Glare.

It is more common in males, between 30 and 50 years of age; the familiar history and previous head trauma increase CH probability; 30 to 80% of the patients have sleep apnoea.

**Cluster headache is a serious condition!**

---

[231] Kandel SA, Mandiga P. Cluster Headache. [Updated 2023 Jul 4]. In: StatPearls [Internet]. Treasure Island (FL): StatPearls Publishing; 2024 Jan-. Available from: https://www.ncbi.nlm.nih.gov/books/NBK544241/

5. The bad sounds of Sleep

The sounds possibly produced during sleep are multiple and varied.

Talking and laughing cand extend crying and screaming. Screaming may have different modalities, from current screams, to piercing screams or to animal-like sounds, such as barking or howling.

Snoring may have quite different intensities and frequencies. 4 types are recognized: Type 1: A low-frequency single syllable snore; Type 2: Duplex sounds that have both low and middle frequencies; Type 3: Duplex sounds that have both low and high frequencies; Type 4: Triplex sounds that have low, middle and high frequencies[232].

Groaning is like a motorbike. Laryngospasm produces a terrible noise.

Bruxism, the "witches" noise

There are possible noises with the mouth, sucking, teeth-chattering, etc

At last, there are the noises of machines to help sleep, such as PAP machines.

---

[232] Snoring sounds and their types (mymed.com)

PEOPLE TELL ME I SNORE

I sleep very well. Sleeping comes easy to me.

I go to bed and zap - in fact, I had already fallen asleep on the sofa and didn't see the Champion's League match - I fell asleep after the first goal, but now the truth is that I am tired.

My head hurts in the morning when I get up. It's a weight that gradually goes away as I get myself ready. But I am tired. I should work less.

The other day I fell asleep during a meeting. It was so embarrassing. The boss banged the table to wake me up. They were discussing the market strategy for the next 6 months and I was snoring.

Sometimes I can even hear myself snoring when I am falling asleep. Liz complains, but I am sure that everybody snores.

I don't understand why I must go to the Doctor.

She says that she can't sleep, and that it is scary to watch me sleeping because I stop breathing and then make these big snorts.

I think I sleep very well, but I have high blood pressure.

High blood pressure and cholesterol. It's this blasted age thing.

Go on a diet, the Doctor says. How is that possible with my working life, the frenzy and lunches with the clients? It's just not on!

Liz has threatened to change rooms. Well, do that then. It's nobody's fault that they snore.

In fact, I've been tired and less up for it.

With the stress at work, it's not possible to have strength for other things.

But the other day things were just not going right. I almost did not manage it. Do you think she noticed?

I am tired.

Liz is always nagging — "you've got to go to the doctor", "it's dangerous for you to drive".

Come again?

I've always been in full control when driving, but the other day I nodded off and went off the road. I woke up with Liz screaming. She was as white as a sheet.

What a drag! Perhaps she is right, and I should go to the doctor.

This patient probably has sleep apnoea because, besides snoring, he has the characteristic symptoms of the condition. Often, since the patient doesn't ear his own snoring, he doesn't assume he/ she really snores.

Classically Sleep apnoea affected 4 to 5% of the adult male population and 2 to 3% of the female. Recent data point to prevalence values much higher: 32.8%: 46.6% in men and 30.5% in women (Tufik et al 2010) and 23.4% in women and 49.7% in men (Heinzer et al 2015).

Apnoea is a pause in breathing. During apnoea the heart beats more slowly, the oxygen in the blood lowers and there is an increase of pressure in the thorax and in the abdomen. The apnoea is resolved with a temporary awakening, which is linked to a snore, to a tachycardia and a temporary increase in blood pressure.

As a result of multiple awakenings, sleep becomes fragmented and light. The patient, despite having the sensation of sleeping, is always waking up without realizing this.

As such, this is a serious problem which must be treated, since it has negative effects on the health of patients. In effect, there are cardiovascular risks (high blood pressure, cardiac problems, strokes, etc.).

There is a high percentage of road accidents due to sleepiness in patients with apnoeas.

Besides these risks, the quality of life is worsened due to the incapacities associated with daily sleepiness and the matrimonial conflicts related to snoring.

Daily sleepiness is often incipient. It seems "natural" to fall asleep watching television, and sometimes it even feels good to fall asleep on the sofa, but the problem becomes clear when the patient is incapable of watching a programme that he/she wants to see. Sleepiness also comes into other aspects of life, during conversations, after meals, in monotonous situations, in public places and in situations which require attention, such as at work and in driving an automobile. Sleepiness is therefore very dangerous.

Matrimonial conflicts frequently involve snoring. Firstly, the couple separates beds, then rooms, and sometimes even partnership, since it is very difficult to sleep beside a snorer. Sometimes it has to do with falling asleep during family conversations or with a lack of libido and sexual capacity which is often an associated feature.

Patients often have an incorrect perception of their problems and often even think that they "sleep very well" due to the ease they have in falling asleep. However, a more detailed analysis shows that they wake with a dry mouth, with a slight headache, are tired and start having memory problems. In fact, sleep apnoea has cognitive risks, with reduction also in executive capacities.

Some patients however have insomnia, especially women.

At night patients get up to urinate and remember their dreams. Some patients also have stomach problems and difficulties in hearing. Many patients are obese or have a large neck and increased waist diameter.

The ingestion of alcoholic drinks is common, but both these and sleeping pills are absolutely contraindicated after dinner in patients with apnoeas.

Comorbidities are common: Hypertension, cardiac arrhythmias, excessive weight or obesity, diabetes or metabolic syndrome, hypercholesterolemia, stroke, cognitive and memory impairment, sexual dysfunction, oesophageal reflux, accidents.

The comorbidity between Sleep apnea and insomnia is referred as COMISA (COMorbid Insomnia and Sleep Apnea)[233], which is associated with impairment of sleep, daytime function, mental health and physical health outcomes, and a higher mortality risk.

The AASM "strongly recommends" for OSAS diagnosis specific rules[234]:

- *Polysomnography (in Lab), or home sleep apnea testing with a technically adequate device, for the diagnosis of OSA in uncomplicated adult patients*
- *Polysomnography (in Lab) should be used for the diagnosis of OSA in patients with significant cardiorespiratory disease, neuromuscular condition, awake or sleep*

---

[233] Sweetman A, Osman A, Lack L, Crawford M, Wallace D. Co-morbid insomnia and sleep apnea (COMISA): recent research and future directions. Curr Opin Pulm Med. 2023 Nov 1;29(6):567-573. doi: 10.1097/MCP.0000000000001007. Epub 2023 Aug 29. PMID: 37642477.

[234] Kapur VK, Auckley DH, Chowdhuri S, Kuhlmann DC, Mehra R, Ramar K, Harrod CG. Clinical Practice Guideline for Diagnostic Testing for Adult Obstructive Sleep Apnea: An American Academy of Sleep Medicine Clinical Practice Guideline. J Clin Sleep Med. 2017 Mar 15;13(3):479-504. doi: 10.5664/jcsm.6506. PMID: 28162150; PMCID: PMC5337595.

hypoventilation, chronic opioid medication use, history of stroke or severe insomnia.

- *If a single home sleep apnea test is negative, inconclusive, or technically inadequate, polysomnography should be performed*
- *Clinical tools, questionnaires and prediction algorithms should not be used to diagnose OSA*

Treatment modalities depend on apnea severity, comorbidities and age. In all cases it involves general measures, and specific treatments with CPAP machine (See "The CPAP changed my life") and Non-CPAP treatments (See "I don't like the machine").

Losing weight is important, and sometimes the loss of a few kilos is enough to obtain beneficial effects. In fact, the loss of weight may lead to curing the problem or be an important support for the other therapeutic measures.

If you suffer from apnoea, treat it before it gets too late.

MY HUSBAND CANNOT STAND MY NOISE

She

I do not believe him; I really think that he is saying that just to pull my leg; I am sure I do not snore since I shared the hotel room with a colleague during a congress and she was not annoyed.

Either he is too sensitive, or we are having a matrimonial crisis. Indeed, the problem is nowadays impacting our 25-year marriage, and we risk divorce.

I come here to ask you some counselling.

He

She snores a lot and you know, as I go to bed late when she is already asleep, I simply cannot stand the noise. Sometimes I get furious, but most of the nights I go to the living room and sleep at the coach. My back is complaining, and my humour is not famous. With all that noise, sex is out of question, and as she does not believe our relations are quite tense. Anything or any small matter ends up in shouting against each other.

Women do not like to snore, since they feel snoring is a male business

The problem is that women, premenopausal and mostly after menopause with ageing and weight gain, often start snoring[235,236]. However, the problem for females is not only snoring but mostly the associated sleep apnoea. Women can have sleep apnoea, just

[235] Heinzer, R., Marti-Soler, H., Marques-Vidal, P., Tobback, N., Andries, D., Waeber, G., ... Haba-Rubio, J. (2018). *Impact of sex and menopausal status on the prevalence, clinical presentation, and comorbidities of sleep-disordered breathing. Sleep Medicine, 51, 29–36.* doi:10.1016/j.sleep.2018.04.016

[236] Perger E, Mattaliano P, Lombardi C. Menopause and Sleep Apnea. Maturitas. 2019 Jun;124:35-38. doi: 10.1016/j.maturitas.2019.02.011. Epub 2019 Feb 28. PMID: 31097176.

like men with a somewhat lower prevalence (1 to 2%); furthermore, they get apnoea at higher Body Mass Indexes than men do, BUT, both snoring and apnoea for females have higher cardiovascular risks than for males[235], therefore the problem is serious and must be treated.

Women with normal BMI might snore due to the upper airway configuration. In these cases, for moderate or mild OSAS, mandibular advancement devices and/or ENT treatments are recommended.

Women have, more often than men an association between OSAS, hypertension and depression and OSAS and insomnia.

When women are overweight and have a moderate or severe apnoea they must use CPAP. Again, some gender differences are possible: a reasonable percentage of women does not stand the CPAP, eventually because the device endangers the female role. Now adays the CPAP machines adjusted for females (CPAP for Her) reduced significantly CPAP rejection.

In this couple snoring is a serious cause for dispute and indeed, whatever the snorer gender, heavy snoring is a possible divorce trigger.

Snoring and sleep apnea are less frequent but more serious in women

THE CPAP CHANGED MY LIFE

You know I love this machine, and I cannot sleep without it.

It changed my life ... before I was not living always tired, always sleepy, forgetting important issues ... I escaped from a terrible accident because my guardian angel protected me, him or someone else ...

You can imagine, I came out the road, asleep of course, and the car went straight downhill in between trees and bushes and stopped 100 meters (330 feet) afterwards because there was a lot of mud and water, whatever ...

I broke my arm, hurt the knee and the leg but nothing serious

Nowadays I take the CPAP everywhere, during travels, holidays and weekends. I use at night and during the naps, whenever possible.

My wife tells me that I am young again ... a very good achievement since these "skills" were forgotten ... you see what I mean ...

The work goes prima.

I don't fall asleep while driving.

Memory seems OK, I might forget people's names, but everybody does.

With the machine I don't snore and the wife is happy.

What better? It is my girlfriend, faithful and always present when needed; we don't argue with each other, and I treat it with great care.

Currently, the most effective treatment consists of the use of a device to sleep, which, in sending pressured air, avoids apnoeas. The pressure may be continuous (CPAP), adjusted to the needs of the patient (APAP), or adjusted to the inspiratory and expiratory pressure levels (BiPAP).

CPAP means continuous positive airway pressure. The pressure is usually applied via a mask placed at the nose (nasal CPAP), at the nose and mouth (facial mask) or with nasal prongs or dream ware placed at the nostrils.

There are basically two types of PAP machines: those that deliver a fixed pressure, which must be set at the level required to maintain the patency of the superior aerial tract, the so-called CPAP machines; and those that automatically calculate the pressure required for that specific patient and that specific apnoea, called APAP machine. It is nowadays consensual that CPAP/APAP machines provide a better long-term protection of the cardiovascular risks of sleep apnoea.

THE AASM recommends the use of both[237]. It must be said that APAP allows home titration.

The good practice statements of the AASM imply: 1) CPAP treatment must be based in diagnostic procedures with objective testing of sleep apnoea; 2) Follow up to solve problems end monitor adherence is required[237].

The CPAP treatment is recommended as first line treatment in patients with moderate or severe sleep apnoea, with marked daytime sleepiness, with impaired sleep related quality of life, with comorbid hypertension[237] with significant medical comorbidities, namely cardio or cerebrovascular[237,238].

---

[237] Patil SP, Ayappa IA, Caples SM, Kimoff RJ, Patel SR, Harrod CG. Treatment of Adult Obstructive Sleep Apnea with Positive Airway Pressure: An American Academy of Sleep Medicine Clinical Practice Guideline. J Clin Sleep Med. 2019 Feb 15;15(2):335-343. doi: 10.5664/jcsm.7640. PMID: 30736887; PMCID: PMC6374094.

[238] Mehrtash M, Bakker JP, Ayas N. Predictors of Continuous Positive Airway Pressure Adherence in Patients with Obstructive Sleep Apnea. Lung. 2019 Apr;197(2):115-121. doi: 10.1007/s00408-018-00193-1. Epub 2019 Jan 7. PMID: 30617618.

A good PAP treatment adaptation implies a regular compliance (usage in more than 70% of the days for more than 4 hours per day)[237]; but it is conventionally accepted that using something is better for the health than not using at all.

PAP treatment has another big advantage: benefits start upon the first day of usage.

Whenever patients adapt well to PAP treatment they feel immediate benefits in their main complaints, sleepiness, vigilance, fatigue, concentration, memory, sexual performance and performance in general. Therefore, severe patients feel their live is "good" again.

Several side effects exist dry nose and mouth, mask leak, mouth leak, nasal congestion, skin lesions around the mask, allergies, air swallowing with flatulence, awakening with machine noise and excessive flow, air flow too cold, air flow affecting the eyes, air flow affecting the bedpartner.

Adherence predictors are however many and include: age (lower in young and in old adults), gender (lower in females), race/ethnicity (eventually lower in African Americans), socioeconomic status (who earn more than average have increased odds of CPAP adherence), smoking status (smokers have lower adherence), severity of OSA (increase adherence), severity of symptoms (increase adherence), social support and bed partner support (increase adherence), Side effects (may decrease adherence)[238].

Patient education, supportive and behavioural interventions play important roles in improving CPAP adherence)[238].

There is no description of CPAP dependence, but its need remains stable in case the patient does not lose weight or does not correct any other sleep apnoea cause.

The CPAP machine performance, compliance and adjustment must be evaluated regularly, together with patients' health status, namely hypertension, body weight, alcoholic beverages consumption, medications affecting sleep related breathing, etc; however, many patients feeling well with the machine do not make any control for many years.

CPAP is good! CPAP makes good!

I DON'T LIKE THE "MACHINE"

I have come here because I cannot bear that thing on my face. I don't get enough air. It seems like I'm suffocating.

I have taken dozens of masks home, tried them all, and I can't stand it. The technicians from the equipment manufacturer were very nice and had a lot of patience. It's just I can't bear them, not the normal ones and not the others which they just put in the nostrils, and not the ones for the nose and for the mouth, none of them. I can tell you, I can't stand any of them.

If I follow their advice and tighten them, they hurt me and I get abrasions on my forehead and on my face. Well abrasions, perhaps not, because I took them off before that happened, but everything went red.

If I don't tighten them, then wind comes to the eyes, which bothers me, and the other day I woke up with my eye all red.

They've told me I must keep my mouth closed, but I can't close my mouth, because my nostrils are blocked, and I can only breathe through my mouth.

And then the air from the contraption is very cold. My nose runs, with the allergy that it causes.

What is more, my wife can't stand it, neither the noise from the device, nor the cold air it lets out. She even came down with a cold.

I continue to feel sleepy, and my wife tells me that I keep on snoring. Sleeping is what bothers me most, but not always. Some days are worse.

I have brought the reading card of the device and what is written here that I am not using it half an hour a night. It and I just don't get along.

I think it is better to give it back and try something else.

Get thinner?

No. You know it's difficult. I have so many dinners out and work lunches. It's impossible to get thinner.

Stop drinking alcoholic beverages? How? In business, wine is good to round off things. I can't be with clients and not join them in a glass of good wine.

What shall I do?

This patient has some complaints related to the side effects of the CPAP machine: Suffocation from the mask, being disturbed, air leaks, abrasions on the face and conjunctivitis. The device is not well accepted by his spouse. Adherence predictors were discussed in the previous chapter [238].

The leaks and the mask must be well corrected and adjusted, but when patients have a nasal obstruction, it is difficult for them to close their mouth. Nasal surgery or medical correction of the problem is advisable.

When a patient cannot stand CPAP, general measures, physiotherapy modalities, mandibular advancement devices (MAD) and ENT or maxillofacial surgeries, hypoglossal stimulation, and sleep apnea medication should be considered and discussed on a case-by-case basis in a multidisciplinary team[239].

Sleep hygiene, lighter dinner not close to bedtime, losing weight and abstain for alcoholic beverages at dinner and before bedtime are highly recommended. Small weight loses have a quite positive impact upon sleep apnoea and together with physical activity they

[239] Arachchige MA, Steier J. Beyond Usual Care: A Multidisciplinary Approach Towards the Treatment of Obstructive Sleep Apnoea. Front Cardiovasc Med. 2022 Jan 5;8:747495. doi: 10.3389/fcvm.2021.747495. PMID: 35071340; PMCID: PMC8767108.

promote health and wellbeing. Measures aiming exercises and other airway training (singing, didgeridoo, instrument playing) that

target oral cavity and oropharyngeal structures may be useful in OSA treatment[240], while mixing amusement features that improve mental health.

General measures are vital, and a lot must be invested in patient behavioural changes.

Positional therapy is particularly important in patients with positional apnoea in supine position; there are devices that render supine position uncomfortable (i.e. the use of tennis ball or equivalent) and electronic devices may alert the supine position by vibration and therefore induce position change, while monitoring objectively patient position.

Positional therapy is better accepted by young people and alone may be insufficient.

Obese patients should raise the headboard to improve breathing during sleep.

Myofunctional therapy (MT) and tongue positioning aiming to strengthen upper airway musculature is quite important[240]. MT provides a reduction in AHI in approximately 50% in adults and 62% in children. The pre and post-MT AHI for adults decreased from 24.5 ± 14.3/h to 12.3 ± 11.8/h, (P < 0.0001) and for paediatric patients, the pre- and post-MT AHI decreased from 4.87 ± 3.0/h to 1.84 ± 3.2/h, P = 0.004.

Drug-induced sleep endoscopy (DISE) should be used whenever it is important to define at which level of the Upper airway occurs

---

[240] Camacho M, Certal V, Abdullatif J, Zaghi S, Ruoff CM, Capasso R, Kushida CA. Myofunctional Therapy to Treat Obstructive Sleep Apnea: A Systematic Review and Meta-analysis. Sleep. 2015 May 1;38(5):669-75. doi: 10.5665/sleep.4652. PMID: 25348130; PMCID: PMC4402674.

the obstruction during an apnoea episode. The ERS has defined both procedures and recommendations[241]

Dentistry treatment involves placing devices to advance the mandible, the lower maxillary bone. Oral devices are first line treatment for primary snoring, for light or moderate apnoeas without somnolence and comorbidities and for patient's intolerant to CPAP[242]. *Main recommendations are:*

Prescription for adult patients who request treatment of primary snoring

Implemented by a qualified dentist who should use a custom, titratable appliance

Follow-up sleep testing to improve or confirm treatment efficacy

The probability of not being able to tolerate a mandibular advancement device after not having tolerated CPAP is higher and should be taken into consideration.

ENT and mandibular surgery have precise indications and, in certain cases, are strongly recommended. There are also other surgical and dentistry treatments.

Amongst the former there are ENT surgical procedures, tonsillectomy and uvulopalatopharyngoplasty (UPPP). Tonsillectomy is recommended in children and adults with

[241] De Vito A, Carrasco Llatas M, Ravesloot MJ, Kotecha B, De Vries N, Hamans E, Maurer J, Bosi M, Blumen M, Heiser C, Herzog M, Montevecchi F, Corso RM, Braghiroli A, Gobbi R, Vroegop A, Vonk PE, Hohenhorst W, Piccin O, Sorrenti G, Vanderveken OM, Vicini C. European position paper on drug-induced sleep endoscopy: 2017 Update. Clin Otolaryngol. 2018 Dec;43(6):1541-1552. doi: 10.1111/coa.13213. Epub 2018 Sep 30. PMID: 30133943.
[242] Ramar K, Dort LC, Katz SG, Lettieri CJ, Harrod CG, Thomas SM, Chervin RD. Clinical Practice Guideline for the Treatment of Obstructive Sleep Apnea and Snoring with Oral Appliance Therapy: An Update for 2015. J Clin Sleep Med. 2015 Jul 15;11(7):773-827. doi: 10.5664/jcsm.4858. PMID: 26094920; PMCID: PMC4481062.

enlarged tonsils. ENT surgery implies the existence of a clearly defined obstruction in the transition between the oropharynx and the nasopharynx and may be carried out for snoring disorders and light apnoea, in children or relatively young adults, and on individuals who are not obese.

Existing studies show that the success of UPPP besides being around 50%, is strongly connected to the surgeon; it should only be used when obstruction caused by OSA is limited to the oropharyngeal

area only[243]. Rhinoplasty can also be considered which can be carried out when there is marked difficulty in the passage of air through the nostrils due to nasal asymmetries.

Maxillofacial surgical interventions have the aim of increasing the antero-posterior diameter of the mandible and are indicated in cases involving the malformation of the face and the lower maxillary bone. This procedure is invasive and requires approval from a variety of clinicians, not the least the maxillofacial surgeon[243].

Hypoglossal nerve electrical stimulation is an emerging OSA treatment. It can be an invasive approach involving the implantation of a neurostimulator in an infraclavicular subcutaneous pocket which delivers an electric current to the distal branch of the hypoglossal nerve or a non-invasive approach to deliver electrical current to the hypoglossal nerve with for instance TESLA devices[200]

Drug Therapy is not recommended for OSA treatment[243]. At present modafinil may be prescribed in patients with sleepiness despite adequate CPAP use. However, several medications are

---

[243] Randerath W, Verbraecken J, de Raaff CAL, Hedner J, Herkenrath S, Hohenhorst W, et al. European Respiratory Society guideline on non-CPAP therapies for obstructive sleep apnoea. Eur Respir Rev. (2021) 30:210200. doi: 10.1183/16000617.0200-2021

emerging as possible solutions[239], namely, Pitolisant hydrochloride (a histamine H3-receptor anatagonist) and Solriamfetol (a dopamine and noradrenaline reuptake inhibitor) used to treat excessive daytime sleepiness, Atomoxetine plus Oxybutinin (Ato-Oxy) combination which has been shown to reduce OSA severity by improving upper airway collapsibility, increasing breathing stability, and augmenting the threshold for arousal in OSA[239].

Any of these types of treatment should only be instigated after a diagnosis of apnoea has been confirmed using a nocturnal polysomnography.

Short- and long-term therapeutic success for excessive somnolence and health risks prevention is certainly greater with ventilation therapy (CPAP).

When you can't bear the "device" there are other actions or treatments which can be carried out. It is essential to do something!

HE SOUNDS LIKE A MOTORBIKE

"I'm not complaining of anything, but she is. Tell her what it's about."

"Well, Doctor, this is not snoring, it's an unbearable grunting, a noise that he starts to make in the early morning, but not always, and for certain periods. Sometimes it stops then, after a while it restarts – I've timed it using my watch – 20 minutes of that and I just can't sleep. It all starts up again about an hour later.

I have tried waking him up but nothing. He's like a stone. He opens his eyes after a while, says something and then goes back to sleep peacefully and starts making that noise again.

Elbowing him doesn't help. He makes the noise whatever position he is in.

I'm telling you doctor it's unbearable. I feel like I am sleeping with an engine!

This noise corresponds to a syndrome called Sleep Related Groaning[244,245]. It is an expiratory REM sleep noise, like a motorbike.

The wife of the patient described some of the characteristics of REM sleep: it occurs at the end of the night, in episodes spaced out in time, of around 1 hour, which last for 20 or 30 minutes.

The noise is not like that of snoring, which is generally sensitive to changes of position. In this case there is no relation to position or to sleep apnoea.

---

[244] American Academy of Sleep Medicine. ICSD-3—International Classification of Sleep Disorders. American Academy of Sleep Medicine, Chicago, 2014

[245] Oldani A, Manconi M, Zucconi M, Castronovo V, Ferini-Strambi L. 'Nocturnal groaning': just a sound or parasomnia? J Sleep Res. 2005 Sep;14(3):305-10. doi: 10.1111/j.1365-2869.2005.00460.x. PMID: 16120106.

Confirmation with polysomnography along with good audio recording equipment is however necessary to confirm the diagnosis.

There is no standardized treatment.

Sleep noises may be strange and not all of them are snoring.

6. SLEEPING TOO MUCH

Sleeping too much is not laziness. It may be due to a characteristic, being a long sleeper, and then it within the normal limits, or to a neurologic dysfunction, a hypersomnia.

Hypersomnias are caused by dysfunction in the Central Nervous System, neurologic or psychiatric.

They are therefore organic and serious disorders

SLEEPINESS IS NOT LAZINESS

"I sleep too much, and I fall asleep easily. It started long ago in my thirties. My family is always making jokes about it. Recently I felt asleep during a party, I was dancing with my husband and zuuut .... a slow dance, a little bit of alcohol, dimmed light, tired and somewhat supported by him ... the perfect climate for an irresistible sleep ... he was furious saying that I don't care for any romance or tenderness between us.

In fact it is an imperious thing which I cannot resist, but it is not always like that, sometimes sleep is more natural, I sleep a little bit and then I am fresh and awake.

The problem is that my nights are terrible I don't sleep well. I thought for some time that the bad nights were making me sleepy during the day. Nowadays I know it is not true since I did not improve with insomnia medication.

They say I am depressed. Of course I am depressed, I don't feel well, I feel a lot of constraints, I don't like jokes around my sleep. My life has a poor quality and nobody understands me."

The prevalence of Excessive Daytime Sleepiness (EDS) in US adults is 33% and in 45% of US adolescents; EDS with symptoms of functional impairment have been found in 15.6% of the general adult population[246].

Sleepiness is not laziness, since it results either from sleep deprivation or circadian misalignment in healthy subjects, from a sleep, medical or psychiatric disorder or from medication.

---

[246] Gandhi KD, Mansukhani MP, Silber MH, Kolla BP. Excessive Daytime Sleepiness: A Clinical Review. Mayo Clin Proc. 2021 May;96(5):1288-1301. doi: 10.1016/j.mayocp.2020.08.033. Epub 2021 Apr 9. Erratum in: Mayo Clin Proc. 2021 Oct;96(10):2729. doi: 10.1016/j.mayocp.2021.08.002. PMID: 33840518.

Patients that suffer from excessive daytime sleepiness are often not understood and joking about it is silly and cruel.

This is true for all ages. A sleepy child must be carefully observed, idem for adolescents, adults and elderly.

Sleepiness is dangerous. Falling asleep involuntarily means that, at this moment, the sleepy persons will not be able to deal with the attitudes required for survival or for efficient communication with others.

It may be the cause of car accidents which the driver is unable to prevent. It may cause attention lapses in a child in the classroom. It may be the cause of catastrophic accidents as many unfortunately reported. It may induce small dramas in daily life like sleeping at the working place, missing a train in the train station, falling asleep in a professional meeting, missing a talk in friends' parties, missing the wife recommendations when watching TV. It may be associated with medical errors[246], etc. etc. etc.

The superficial way society often envisages sleepiness leads frequently to marked delays in diagnosis.

Sleepiness is irresistible and sleep attacks impend upon vigilance in a sudden and unexpected way.

This case history does not allow any diagnosis, and a more detailed anamnesis is required and also some laboratorial test, namely at least Polysomnography (PSG), Multiple Sleep Latency test (MSLT) and Actigraphy.

- *In case Actigraphy reveals adequate sleep schedules and sleep duration and the MSLT confirms excessive sleepiness and REM sleep abnormalities the patient has a Narcolepsy without cataplexy or Narcolepsy type 2.*
- *In case Actigraphy reveals inadequate sleep schedules and/or reduced sleep duration patient has inadequate*

sleep hygiene, which must be corrected before any further evaluation.

- *In case PSG reveals either sleep apnoea, upper airway resistance syndrome, periodic limb movements of sleep or any other abnormality which would cause daytime sleepiness, than these would be the proper diagnosis.*
- *In case Actigraphy reveals a sleep phase delay syndrome this possibility should be considered*
- *In case the patient has a medical, or a neurological or a psychiatric disorder they should be considered in the context of excessive daytime sleepiness.*

Excessive daytime sleepiness is a serious problem in all ages

REALLY OUT OF IT

"Tony, come here. I am worried. Alex isn't waking up. I've shaken him, yelled, taken his jim jams off, opened the window - nothing. He gives a kind of grunt and just carries on sleeping. It seems like it's the same as it was a few months back."

"Alex get up, it's 10 o'clock."

"Er. Er. Alright, I'm awake. Keep your hair on."

"There he goes, straight for the fridge."

"It's just like the other time when he cleaned out the fridge. Alex, you're sleeping on your feet. Don't walk through the house naked."

"Leave me alone."

"Don't eat any more. Tony, get ready. We're taking him to the Hospital again."

"They didn't find anything last time. They did a CT scan, MRI, Lumbar Puncture, everything normal. Do you want to do that all again? The puncture was no joke."

"Look, he's just eaten 5 bread rolls, 3 yoghurts, the rest of the chicken from yesterday and a litre of milk. What should we do?"

"Don't be silly, Alex and behave. Get a hold of yourself please. This is your mother, mind your manners. You can still be slapped."

"Leave him alone. Go to bed again. Go and sleep until tomorrow."

This situation, with recurrent episodes which last for several days, of hypersomnia (sleeping more than 14 hours a day), hyperphagia (eating too much) and being sexually uninhibited, constitute Kleine-Levin syndrome[247] or recurrent hypersomnia.

---

[247] Shah F, Gupta V. Kleine-Levin Syndrome (KLS) [Updated 2023 Aug 8]. In: StatPearls [Internet]. Treasure Island (FL): StatPearls Publishing; 2024 Jan-. Available from: https://www.ncbi.nlm.nih.gov/books/NBK568756/

It is a rare disorder, 1 to 5 cases per million population, occurring mostly in male adolescents, recurrently, with completely normal sleep and behaviour in the intervals.

This results from a dysfunction of the diencephalon, namely the hypothalamus, the area of the brain which controls sleep and appetite, and the episodes terminate spontaneously. Possible aetiologies include a psychologic disturbance, trauma, toxins, infection, serotonergic or dopaminergic neurotransmitter abnormalities, and autoimmunity[247].

Symptoms include hypersomnia, cognitive abnormalities (confusion, concentration, attention, temporal disorientation, altered perception and memory defects, such as, amnesia), speech difficulties (mutism and slurred speech), eating behaviours (hyperphagia, sweets preference), depressive mood with possible suicidal ideation, hypersexuality (sexual advances, masturbation, exposing oneself and obscene language), compulsive behaviours (singing, writing, body rocking, chewing one's lips)[247].

Due to the somnolence and the behavioural alterations, this may be confused with encephalitis.

Diagnosis is made by taking the clinical history. Sleep monitoring over a 24-hour period confirms the typical alterations in sleep.

The patient is spontaneously cured after some time, but there is specific treatment for the hypersomnia episodes.

There is specific treatment with wakefulness stimulants, similar to those used in Narcolepsy, carbamazepine, or Lithium.

Recurrent hypersomnia is a specific disorder. It is typical of male adolescents.

I SPEND MY LIFE SLEEPING

You know, my problem is that I sleep a lot. I mean, I need a lot of hours of sleep.

When I sleep less than 11, 12 hours, I spend the day sleepy.

I really must have a nap, otherwise I am drunk with sleepiness and do not know what I am doing.

My family just does not understand. They think it's all crazy and everything is just a sign of laziness. That I don't want to do very much and that I don't like my job.

It's not true. I really try to do everything well and I don't make any mistakes or get behind in my work.

What is certain is that I have 4 or 5 fewer hours in the day than others, and as a result I cannot do as much.

There's a long history of anger, exchanges and banter in my family with regard to my sleeping.

There was a time when they thought it was all psychological, but it certainly isn't the case that I am depressed, although it is annoying the way they deal with this.

There was also a time when they tried everything — alarm clocks, radios, phones, ice on my face, slapping me, whatever... but as they never managed to wake me up after 8 hours of sleep, they gave up.

Now I live alone to avoid any more exchanges or conflicts.

I am adapting as much as I can, and I have my life more or less organized.

"Do you sleep well?"

"At night yes, the sleep is quite long."

"And are you sleepy during the day?"

"Not if I sleep all those hours... I mean... sometimes I feel a little bit sleepy if I'm being honest, but not always. Do you think there is a solution?"

The patient, after ruling out cataplexy, hypnagogic hallucinations, sleep paralysis and family history, probably has hypersomnia with increased total sleep, Idiopathic Hypersomnia (IH)[248].

The complaints are real, the situation is serious and must be diagnosed through hormonal examinations, to rule out hypothyroidism, brain imaging tests to rule out neurological alterations, a polysomnography and a multiple sleep latency test which will rule out narcolepsy and an actigraphy to prove the excess in total sleep.

Idiopathic hypersomnia is characterized by excessive daytime sleepiness, uncontrollable need to sleep with long unrefreshing naps, and difficulty waking up from sleep in most instances despite average or longer amounts of nocturnal sleep for at least three months[249].

It is a rare disorder with no gender differences. The prevalence increased in the last decade by 32% (from 7.8 to 10.3 per 100,000 persons)[248].

The pathophysiology IH remains unknown.

The symptoms are long daytime non-refreshing naps (>1 hour); there are 2 subtypes concerning sleep duration, which can be long (longer than 10h) and short sleep duration. Furthermore, patients may have severe sleep inertia, fatigue, and evening chronotype

[248] Dhillon K, Sankari A. Idiopathic Hypersomnia. [Updated 2023 Jul 31]. In: StatPearls [Internet]. Treasure Island (FL): StatPearls Publishing; 2024 Jan-. Available from: https://www.ncbi.nlm.nih.gov/books/NBK585065/

[249] American Academy of Sleep Medicine. ICSD-3—International Classification of Sleep Disorders. American Academy of Sleep Medicine, Chicago, 2014

tendency, and also brain fog, and sleep drunkenness in IH with long sleep duration; automatic behaviours, sleep paralysis, and hypnogogic hallucinations may also occur [248].

The social and familial implications are obvious, but these cases are as organic as any other disorder; making fun of them is absurd and nasty.

Treatment is complex and involves sleep hygiene rules and the use of wakefulness stimulants. Modafinil is considered the first-line treatment option. Oxibate, amphetamines and Pitolisant are other possible options

__Idiopathic hypersomnia is a serious and debilitating condition.__

I SPEND THE DAY LYING DOWN SLEEPING

My problem is that I am always sleepy. At night, daytime, I spend all my time in bed. I get up late, I go to bed early, in the afternoon I go and lie down because I am very tired and I have to sleep.

The more I sleep, the sleepier I am.

You want to know what time I get up?... between midday and 1:00 pm

And what time I have a nap? Around 4:00 pm to 7:00 pm. At 10:00 pm I'm already in bed and I sleep until the morning.

How does everything work at home? Well, badly, of course. I can't do a lot and neither do I feel like doing so. The arguments are huge, or rather they used to be, because now the silence is total. The ice between us is colder than polar ice.

Children? Yes, I have got a boy and a girl – she has already left home, and he is studying, but his marks are nothing special.

Nobody pays attention to me at home... I am completely alone. Depressed? Well, what do you think? I've thought several times it would be better just to end it all. This is not life. This is nothing.

"You will have to do some tests."

"I am not sure I am able to! Do I have to leave home? It was so difficult just coming here today..."

The exams that the patient must do are similar to those for narcolepsy and the other hypersomnias. Depression scales should be utilised as well as a sleep diary and sleep questionnaires.

In this case, the most probable outcome is to have a polysomnography showing either non-specific alterations or the alterations characteristic of depression, a normal multiple sleep latency test and a high level of depression.

If it is shown that the patient is not sleeping 18 hours a day as she reports, she is probably suffering from depression with hypersomnia[250].

Depression is seen in various psychiatric diseases: major depressive disorder (MDD), bipolar disorder (BD), and seasonal affective disorder (SAD). In these conditions a high frequency of EDS, prolonged nocturnal sleep, and sleep inertia has been reported[250].

MDD has excessive sleep duration (6%), but their sleep duration is lower than Idiopathic hypersomnia, and despite EDS complaints the MSLT values were normal[250].

BD has a higher frequency of hypersomnolence, ranging from 23% to 78%, however excessive sleep duration is in most studies not confirmed with actigraphic measures, but that excessive sleepiness predicts relapse to mania[250].

In SAD hypersomnolence is a major feature with frequencies varying from 67% to 76%, but again objective data are lacking[250].

These cases benefit from complementary phototherapy treatment and anti-depressive treatment.

<u>Depression is a possible cause of hypersomnia.</u>

---

[250] Lopez R, Barateau L, Evangelista E, Dauvilliers Y. Depression and Hypersomnia: A Complex Association. Sleep Med Clin. 2017 Sep;12(3):395-405. doi: 10.1016/j. jsmc.2017.03.016. Epub 2017 May 26. PMID: 28778237.

7. UNREGULATED SLEEP

Don't forget you have clocks in your body and in your brain, real biological clocks which measure time as well as your wristwatch. These watches are a huge biological advantage and don't like to be detuned, if you change your schedule every day, if you do large variations in your bedtime, in getting up or in going to sleep.

In circadian disorders there is a misalignment between the individual endogenous rhythm and the sleep-wake schedule needed for work and social activities, which causes daytime sleepiness and/or insomnia and significant impairment in daily occupational activities

I ALWAYS ARRIVE LATE

I cannot arrive on time.

They are all there waiting for me and here I am again making up a little fib. What will it be today? I've been throwing up? That's it! I have told them so many times there was so much traffic, so today had better be different. They are going to be furious.

I can't fall asleep before 2 a.m., and I can't wake up in the morning. Whatever I do, it doesn't work. I set 2 alarm clocks and my mobile phone, which does not turn off, but I am so sleepy that I turn everything off as sleep is much stronger. These guys are idiots and don't know how to drive. Life sucks.

The clock in the car is 5 minutes fast, or is that 10 minutes? If it was, I'd still have a few minutes.

OK, I vomited... Something that disagreed with me... What excuse am I going to give for arriving late, even after scheduling the meeting for 10:00 am?

10:30 am! What a drag! Of course I can't take the kids to school. Get up at 7:00 am!? I would die.

My husband thinks I am lazy. All I want to do is sleep.

He is like a morning cock and at 7:00 am he is as fresh as a daisy. Not me. I function well at night.

What an idiot, cutting in without looking. If he thinks I'm going to let him get by he's wrong. I can also drive, you cretin.

Ha hah! Of course I overtook the "hair do"!

It's almost 11:00 am. My God...

I'm almost arriving. If only there was a bit less traffic on the main road. I would be there in a jiffy.

I'm alright at night, when I can think clearly, when I have radiant ideas, when I work well. Morning is a horror show. I try and go to bed earlier but I just can't. The doctor gave me some pills, but the one and only time I tried them, I was just zonked. I felt like I had been drugged and I bumped into someone in a traffic jam. A horror show!

Right, here I am. Just need to park the car. God willing there will be a place. Here is not so good, but never mind. Just hope the lift works and it is waiting for me down below.

....

Hi, Good Morning. I am sorry for the delay. It's just, besides the traffic, I had a bad night... I must have eaten something that disagreed with me.

Shall we get started?

When you sleep well, but fall asleep late, at 2:00 am or even later (it can get to 5:00 am or 6:00 am) and you also wake up at 10:00 am or even later at 2:00 pm or 4 :00 pm, this can be considered as being a delay sleep phase syndrome (DSPS)[251,252].

That is, these individuals sleep reasonably well but fall asleep and wake up later.

Falling asleep, sleeping, waking up and being alert during the day follow the body's temperature curve, which, when lower, increases the tendency for sleep and when high increases wakefulness. In these patients, the curve has a normal progression, but everything happens later, this is the sleep phase delay.

---

[251] Narala B, Ahsan M, Ednick M, Kier C. Delayed sleep wake phase disorder in adolescents: an updated review. Curr Opin Pediatr. 2024 Feb 1;36(1):124-132. doi: 10.1097/MOP.0000000000001322. Epub 2023 Dec 6. PMID: 38054481.

[252] Culnan, E., McCullough, L. M., & Wyatt, J. K. (2019). *Circadian Rhythm Sleep-Wake Phase Disorders. Neurologic Clinics.* doi:10.1016/j.ncl.2019.04.003

As such, this is a physiological problem that is not solved through acts of will. In turn, hypnotics have negative effects and do not solve the problem.

These patients are a more serious variation of a spectrum of the normal population which includes daytime and nighttime individuals, that is, the larks and the owls.

In some cases, the situation becomes worse, that is, falling asleep can occur much later, at 6:00 am, for example, and waking up at 4:00 pm. They have an inversion of the sleep wake cycle. This makes most school programmes impossible to carry out or working in most jobs. Only those with nocturnal professions are adapted to this type of biological rhythm.

Delayed sleep wake phase disorder has a range of prevalence between 1% and 16%[251].

Often it is associated with neurodevelopmental disorders (attention deficit hyperactivity disorder and autism spectrum disorder) as well as psychopathology (substance use, anxiety, and depression)[251]. Another common symptom is procrastination, which increasing the tendency to perpetuate negative situations and chieving no solutions.

There is often confusion with insomnia due to the difficulty in falling asleep at earlier hour[252]. In these cases, taking hypnotics aggravates the problem, may induce dependence and is not effective. There are two subtypes of DSPD, those that have really a delayed melatonin DLMO curve, and those who have a normal melatonin DLMO curve but behave as DSPD[253].

---

[253] Reis C, Paiva T. Delayed sleep-wake phase disorder in a clinical population: gender and sub-population diferences. Sleep Sci. 2019 Jul-Sep;12(3):203-213. doi:10.5935/1984-0063.20190086. PubMed PMID: 31890097; PubMed Central PMCID: PMC6932846

The DSPD is not treatable by current therapies. Treatment implies chronotherapy such as progressively increasing/decreasing the sleep onset until an adjusted time is achieved, or the use of ultra-bright light (7000–12,000 lux) in the morning and melatonin (or its derivatives) at night.

A classical chronotherapy procedure sets an individual on a 27-hour sleep-wake schedule, by prescribing bedtime 3 hours later each day; other variants have been used (eg,2-hour delays, twice per week[252].

Light used in the morning makes you fall asleep earlier.

Administering melatonin at night simulates the endogenous production of the hormone with the same name.

If you cannot meet morning schedules don't feel guilty. It's your physiological rhythm.

I GO TO BED VERY EARLY

I like to go to bed early. We have dinner at 6:30, 7:00 pm tops. I go to bed at 8:30 pm. At 9:00 pm, if I am not already asleep, I am dying to sleep. I get up early. Really early! At 4:00 or 4:30 am, at the maximum, I am already awake. I wake up well, without the wish to sleep any more, not tired, nothing.

I think I should go and live in an Amish community. I wouldn't have any problems there, but with so much electricity and so many ads inviting me to go out at night, it's very hard for me to synchronize everything.

I am the first to get to work. At 7:00 am I am there, before everybody else. They had to give me a key, since I operate in a very literal sense like the morning cock. I get everything up and running, and when the others arrive, all the machines and their computers are switched on.

But before arriving I do gymnastics at home, since there aren't any health clubs or swimming pools that open so early.

I organize my life when everybody is still asleep and when the first plane flies over my house, I have already been awake for a long time.

I am always waiting for the shops to open in the morning.

It's at night that I can't do anything. I would make a good farmer or baker. But no, I am a machine technician.

The problem, or maybe it isn't even a problem, is that I am not alone. My wife is not like me, but she goes to bed and gets up relatively early, but the children, the boy and the girl, take after me. At least I won't have to collect them from the pub when they are more grown up. But as I have never seen anybody like this I came to find out if this is normal.

In effect, this is a portrait of an advanced sleep wake phase disorder (ASWPD)[254,255] with familiar characteristics, which is relatively rare.

What this means is that the endogenous temperature rhythm which regulates the sleep-wakefulness cycle and melatonin rhythm are shifted 3 to 4 hours and everything happens earlier, consequently the tendency to fall asleep and wake up also happens earlier[256].

ASWPD may initially appear as if they have a disorder of excessive daytime sleepiness (since they can't stand late parties) or depression (since they wake up too early)[254].

This is an organic problem and the genes responsible for this situation has already been identified, namely, mutations in clock genes Per2, CK1δ, Cry2 and Per3[256]. It is not however clear that all cases are hereditary, but what is certain is that it is a real problem, not controllable through the self-will or determination of individuals.

There is no evidence of melatonin use in the morning in ASWPD. On the days when they must go to bed later, they can avoid problems by exposing themselves to bright light or dim light at the end of the day. Dim light has lower side effects than bright light; nevertheless, the phototherapy side effects are minimal and transient (eyestrain, nausea, agitation, and headaches). This light exposure delays falling asleep and used on special days for parties or night events, can avoid certain unpleasant situations.

Waking up and falling asleep early is a physiological characteristic.

---

[254] Culnan, E., McCullough, L. M., & Wyatt, J. K. (2019). *Circadian Rhythm Sleep-Wake Phase Disorders. Neurologic Clinics.* doi:10.1016/j.ncl.2019.04.003

[255] American Academy of Sleep Medicine. ICSD-3—International Classification of Sleep Disorders. American Academy of Sleep Medicine, Chicago, 2014

[256] Liu C, Tang X, Gong Z, Zeng W, Hou Q, Lu R. Circadian Rhythm Sleep Disorders: Genetics, Mechanisms, and Adverse Effects on Health. Front Genet. 2022 Apr 29;13:875342. doi: 10.3389/fgene.2022.875342. PMID: 35571019; PMCID: PMC9099045.

I TRAVEL A LOT

I am more and more tired, with concentration problems and unable to sleep.

I travel a lot. I live in Moskow, but my family is in Portugal, so I come back every weekend.

My work is quite demanding, and I used to cope well with the work and the travelling, but I start feeling uneasy sometimes, with unwanted sleep during work, difficulty to sleep at night and a mild irritability.

I start forgetting names of persons I should remember which is sometimes quite embarrassing.

I live at a Hotel during the week with all the facilities but I feel alone, especially in the weekends I stay in Moskow. Sometimes I feel a subtle sadness and I got some extra pounds, I and some gastric complaints and most of all I don't feel well.

Nowadays many people have this split type of life. They are abroad and return regularly home where the family remains.

This occurs in officials of political institutions, such as the European Commission or the United Nations, in executives of big multinational enterprises, in pilots or cabin staff of airflight companies, etc, etc.

They are usually highly skilled and highly trained persons, but they must face two problems: the frequent travelling and the recurrent circadian misalignment.

Frequent travelling in executives per se provokes a sleep curtailment; adding to it the sleep reduction and the circadian shifts due to travelling into different time zones, the problem may become serious.

Airline flight crews mix shift work, jetlag and frequent air pressure changes associated with landing and take-off. The have a higher prevalence of fatigue, sleepiness and susceptibility to sleep and mental disorders[257,258]

Some adapt better than others.

Counselling must consider many factors, namely the direction of the shift (to east/ to west/ to North/ to South) and the number of time zones crossed. It is essential to keep "the time" of a specific time zone, maintaining identical schedules whenever possible despite travelling.

Going North or South is associated with climate changes, which also require specific counselling.

Furthermore, the frequency of travelling must be reduced to a "reasonable amount", approaching the "minimum possible", after integration of the familiar needs and work specificities.

At the working place discussion of all the unnecessary stress events must be evaluated, so that stress is reduced. Furthermore, the issues concerning comfort, loneliness, nutrition and regular exercise must be seriously considered and optimized.

At home the same issues must be evaluated, so that conflicts are minimized, unnecessary compensations rationalized, etc.

The objective is to achieve the best possible balance and the best possible quality of life. Furthermore, subtle or obvious signs of a sleep disorder and/or medical or psychological/psychiatric dysfunction must be evaluated and treated.

Keep your preferable time in case you travel a lot

---

[257] Wen, C.C.Y.; Cherian, D.; Schenker, M.T.; Jordan, A.S. Fatigue and Sleep in Airline Cabin Crew: A Scoping Review. Int. J. Environ. Res. Public Health **2023**, 20, 2652. https://doi.org/10.3390/ijerph20032652

[258] Reis C, Mestre C, Canhão H, Paiva T, Gradwell D Sleep and fatigue differences in the two most common types of commercial flight operations Aviat Space Environ Med. 2016, Sep;87(9):811-5.

I AM FLYING EAST, TO LISBON, WHAT SHOULD I DO?

I live in Miami. It is lovely, full of houses of great artists, a kind of natural paradise lost and transformed into a real estate paradise, but still beautiful, with water everywhere, replete with every colour and shape, and a general atmosphere of relaxation and fiesta blessed by a pleasant climate and an ever-present sun.

I travelled to Lisbon to a meeting and some city seeing.

Lisbon is a city with a special sunlight, that blends old-world charm with modern features. From its narrow streets to the iconic yellow trams, from the old monuments and the immense Tagus Estuary, everything is beautiful.

But the trip was awful, so long, hours and hours on the plane. Of course I slept during the journey. When we got there, I didn't even know what time it was, if it was the time from here or from there. But it was late. Everybody was worn out with the transfers, queues and customs and we all went to sleep again. I woke up fresh as a daisy, but I couldn't go back to sleep at local hours.

Next day, I should wake up too early for my usual hours and I was sleep deprived. During a meeting I fell asleep without wanting to. Nodding off with my mouth open was so embarrassing. Next three days I couldn't fit.

I don't like this happening to me, and I would like to know what I should do.

Current air travel at high speed enables various time zones to be crossed passing from the place of origin to other places with many hours of difference. The difference from Miami-Lisbon is 4 hours and the journey to cross the Atlantic takes around 8:30 hours. Therefore, those who leave, for example, at 4:30 pm will arrive at 1:00 am, but locally it will already 5:00 am and those who leave at 0:30 am will arrive at 9:00 am but locally it is around 2pm. This is what is called desynchronization or jet-lag, that is, one's internal biological clock shows a time different from the external or environmental clock.

Flying east is worse than flying west. Journeys to the east make our clock go backwards, and there is a more difficult and lengthy adaptation than in journeys to the west.

Consider that you need 1 day for each hour difference in time zone.

The symptoms of jet-lag or flight dysrhythmia[259] are: Fatigue Insomnia and sleepiness, difficulty with concentration, mood disturbances, lack of appetite and gastrointestinal alterations, and performance difficulties.

You must take these symptoms into account in long airplane travel.

Adaptation depends on the number of time zones travelled and trip purpose and duration. In case your trip duration is shorter than the time zones travelled it is better to keep your original time schedule; in case the trip is longer it is better to adjust to local time.

When you travel east it is recommended that you do the journey at night and sleep during the journey. It is better to choose the night flight of the case story and get the local sunshine upon arrival to adjust.

When you travel west it is recommended that you don't sleep during the flight, and try to sleep later, at the local time, as this increases the pressure to sleep and wake up will be later at an hour closer to that of the place travelled to.

---

[259] Cingi C, Emre IE, Muluk NB. Jetlag related sleep problems and their management: A review. Travel Med Infect Dis. 2018 Jul-Aug;24:59-64. doi: 10.1016/j.tmaid.2018.05.008. Epub 2018 May 19. PMID: 29787851.

There is considerable individual variability in the ability to adapt the circadian rhythm. Night owls adapt better than morning larks.

There are sites which teach you what to do depending on the journey you are making[260] (www.bodyclock.com), but in general terms the travel recommendations are the following:

Before the journey

    Find out information about this issue in advance

    Sleep and rest well before a long-haul flight

During the journey

    Hydrate well

    Reduce your consumption of alcoholic and caffeine drinks

    Light meals

    Adjust your mealtimes to the local arrival time

    Rapid action non-BZD hypnotics on the flight and the first days after arriving (with a medical prescription)

After arriving

    If your dislocation is going to last less than 72 hours it is better not to adjust

    If your dislocation is going to last more than 72 hours you should adjust immediately, eating and absorbing the light at the destination location

    You should avoid important activities (business and competitions) in the first 48 hours

    Rapid action non-BZD hypnotics in the first nights (if necessary)

    Modafinil in the morning in the first few days (if necessary)

    Caffeine

    Morning phototherapy or catch the local sun light

    Melatonin: When taken it should be around 20 hours from the place of arrival for a duration in agreement with the time zone difference (5hours difference 5 days).

---

[260] www.bodyclock.com

There are special recommendations for flights to the east, namely:

Bring the sleep stage forward 3 days previously by 1 to 2 hours per day, with morning light and melatonin in the afternoon

When you travel think about your internal clocks to reduce jet lag.

I AM ADRIFT

It's been like this for years. I just can't adjust my schedule to that of other people.

I cannot wake up at set hours. Some days the alarm clock helps, and others it just doesn't.

Sometimes I function well in the morning and at other times I work better in the afternoon.

I fall asleep during the day just like at night. I feel some sleepiness.

To balance myself I must be incredibly careful: set hours to wake up, to catch the bus, to get to work, to leave work, etc.

Despite these efforts, the result isn't always good.

It's always been like this. It was like this when I was a kid. I remember well my mother's care and her concerns with me.

I have been blind since birth, and despite this I have had a professional life just like the others. Almost like the others, though I think my effort has been greater.

As the circadian system is synchronized by light which stimulates the retina, many visually impaired individuals have great problems in synchronizing to the 24-hour day-night rhythm[261].

The eye is simultaneously a visual organ and a circadian organ. Circadian regulation is achieved through certain special retina cells, the ganglion cells, which are sensitive to the blue light spectrum – that is, different cells of the cones and rods which enable us to see.

---

[261] Hartley S, Dauvilliers Y, Quera-Salva MA. Circadian Rhythm Disturbances in the Blind. Curr Neurol Neurosci Rep. 2018 Aug 6;18(10):65. doi: 10.1007/s11910-018-0876-9. PMID: 30083814.

This means that an individual may be severely visually impaired (blind) and maintain circadian regulation. More frequently both systems are affected.

therefore, visually impaired individuals suffer from major disturbances, such as this patient's which appears to be a circadian "free runner", or eventually having a delayed sleep phase disorder (DSPD), advance sleep phase (ASPD) or a circadian cycle different from 24 hour (N24SWD)[261]*.*

Treatment involves behaviour therapy, sleep scheduling, and the use of melatonin or equivalent, Ramelteon, or in Europe, Circadin or Melatonin.

The visually impaired have sleep disturbances which, often, they don't take seriously.

8. STRANGE BEHAVIOURS DURING SLEEP

During sleep both brain electric activity (EEG) and brain connectivity (brain areas communication) changes according to what is called sleep stages; furthermore, some behaviours such as eating, micturition, are actively inhibited to protect sleep continuity.

During Slow Wave Sleep there is a marked **EEG** slowing and a synchronization of many cortical areas; in case an arousal occurs during this period things might go wrong, and unwanted and involuntary behaviours might occur: screaming, walking around, violence, etc.

We dream more often during **REM** sleep, but we should no do whatever we are dreaming, therefore during **REM** the locomotor system is inhibited; in some pathologies this protective inhibition does not occur, and people is acting out their dreams: violent behaviours might occur. On the other hand, **REM** sleep dreams can be terrifying, and the dreamers wake up in distress.

Eating, micturition, defecation, and sexual activity might occur during sleep

Altogether these behaviours are called "Parasomnias"

I HAVE VIOLENT DREAMS

— You know, I have nowadays strange dreams during which I hurt myself. Some days ago, I dreamed that somebody was trying to steal my car, and I attacked him so violently that I broke the marble of bedside table

— You can't imagine! He hurt himself. His face had several bruises and hematomas, and he didn't broke the nose because he was using the mask of the CPAP machine

— I can show you the photos. Here you see the marble cover without the corner. It is about 1 inch thick! I broke it with my face

— Show your photos! You see the danger. A big damage in his own face.

— Yes, I have sleep apnoea and I use a CPAP machine, but this was during a dream.

— He falls from bed in other occasions, and he often screams and kicks me. I am always watching him afraid something happens

— Yes, in my dreams I am attacked by strangers, once it was an animal, and I must defend myself.

— Even with the CPAP he is never quiet. He moves, jumps, kicks. It is a restless sleep, but the violent episodes occur mostly at dawn, by 5 or 6 am.

These episodes of violence in the older adults in the early morning which result from a dreaming context are REM parasomnias (REM behaviour disorder- RBD)[262].

These individuals, normally of the male sex, and often elders, no longer possess REM sleep motor inhibition (REM atonia) and start

---

[262] Dauvilliers Y, Schenck CH, Postuma RB, Iranzo A, Luppi PH, Plazzi G, Montplaisir J, Boeve B. REM sleep behaviour disorder. Nat Rev Dis Primers. 2018 Aug 30;4(1):19. doi: 10.1038/s41572-018-0016-5. PMID: 30166532.

acting out their dreams. As such, within the context of their dream they will attack anyone who is nearby or hurt themselves in this defensive act.

The episodes are dangerous for them and for their bed partner, since physical lesions are common.

The dangers are multiple: hematomas, trauma, falls, concussions, broken arms, black eyes, etc

During the episodes several behaviours might be observed: talking, laughing, shouting, swearing, gesturing, reaching, grabbing, arm flailing, slapping, kicking, leaping from bed, crawling, running. However, some behaviours never occur in RBD: chewing, feeding, drinking, sexual behaviour, urination and defecation.

These patients are usually quiet and non-aggressive people during the day, and they will feel surprised, guilty and worried with the effects of their acts.

REM behaviour disorder is associated with other disorders but may occur without any other pathology. These episodes can herald the development of dementia and Parkinson disease, occurring many years before. Indeed, there are 3 subtypes: Idiopathic RBD, Drug induced RBD and Secondary RBD due to medical/neurological disease. The associations with periodic limb movements is quite frequent.

Given this, these patients need to be observed by specialists, and sleep tests should be carried out, preferably video-polysomnography along with brain imaging tests (MRI) and cognitive function evaluation.

Treatment is easy and obligatory, with specific drugs such as clonazepam or melatonin, and should be started immediately after a correct diagnosis.

Protection measures are required, namely removing any sharp objects around, covering the floor with pillows, using separate beds or separate rooms whenever convenient, etc.

Nocturnal violence is dangerous, but usually easily treatable.

I HATE DOCTORS

"My head hurts. My head really hurts."

"Well, it happened again tonight, and I am sure you hurt yourself."

"I did! And my arm hurts. What did I do?"

"Don't you remember?"

"No! All I know is my head and my arm hurt. I'm in a hurry."

"Let's see... Your arm is injured all over. You must have hit it against the wall or the door. I'll get the alcohol."

"Not the alcohol, it burns. Get the hydrogen peroxide."

"But you're hurt."

"I am tired. My head hurts."

"Do you want to eat?"

"I'm not hungry, I'm in agony."

"We woke up when you shouted. Your yelling was scary. You were on the bed saying incomprehensible things."

"What time was it?"

"It was 5:00 am You didn't let us sleep and now I am also so tired."

"This is too much. The boy must be treated. Have you seen the state of his arm?"

"I took him to the GP and he requested a battery of tests which came out normal. They said that it cannot be epilepsy because it only happens when sleeping."

"We must look for another doctor. This is weird and dangerous."

"The other day it happened when you were having a nap. Do you remember?"

"He doesn't say anything. He's over there confused. Take an aspirin and your headache will go away."

"I can't go to classes."

"Don't you remember anything?"

"I've already told you, no."

"Take an aspirin and it will go away."

"I'll see if I can take you to a specialist. I'm going to arrange another appointment."

....

"I must tell you that I hate doctors. I don't like them. I don't trust them."

"!?"

"I came here so my conscience is clear, because I don't believe in anything or anyone."

"!!!"

"There are things that happen to me at night. They have said it was epilepsy, they have said it wasn't. What is certain is that it hasn't gone away even with all the treatments. I've been like this for 9 years. It happens 3 or 4 times a night. In the middle of the night."

My tests are normal. CT and MRI."

"What happens?"

"I don't really know. I don't remember. I just know that I hit my arm against the wall. Can you see, I've got scabs on my arms."

"The movement must be really violent for your arm to be like that."

"Yes, it is. I hit my right arm against the wall, and I get worked up. I don't remember anything. I don't bite my tongue. I don't wee. In the morning I'm exhausted. Like I said, this happens every night, three or four times a night."

"Have you done any sleeping tests?"

"No."

"You'll have to do them. I'll schedule a test for tomorrow using video during the night."

This conversation appears to show that the patient has sleep related epilepsy. It is essential to differentiate epileptic seizures from sleep-related paroxysmal events[263].

These episodes, which occur in the middle of the night or in the early morning and start in adolescence, young adulthood or adulthood, are probably not sleepwalking.

Diagnosis is essential since epilepsy requires treatment.

Many aspects are suggestive: only at night and during sleep, different times of the night, repetition of an identical movement, the absence of memory, being exhausted and having headaches the following day.

Diagnosis can be carried out with video polysomnography including 19 EEG channels. This technique enables visualization of both interictal paroxysmal activity (activity occurring in between seizures) and seizures recording.

One third of epilepsies take place exclusively during sleep, and the seizures described in this case may correspond to frontal or

---

[263] Liu WK, Kothare S, Jain S. Sleep and Epilepsy. Semin Pediatr Neurol. 2023 Dec;48:101087. doi: 10.1016/j.spen.2023.101087. Epub 2023 Sep 24. PMID: 38065633.

*temporal epilepsies. **NREM** sleep is a facilitator of seizure activity, while **REM** sleep is a suppressor[264].*

Behavioural patterns during these epileptic seizures are extremely variable, but most patients do not have any recollection of the episodes, or if they do, they are extremely vague. Shouting, sometimes piercing, occurs during epilepsy, night terrors and psychogenic episodes.

Most cases do not run in the families, but there is a form of hereditary frontal epilepsy.

A correct diagnosis and suitable treatment with anticonvulsants to stop the seizures, are essential.

Epilepsy is activated by sleep and seizures may only occur at night.

---

[264] Carreño M, Fernández S. Sleep-Related Epilepsy. Curr Treat Options Neurol. 2016 May;18(5):23. doi: 10.1007/s11940-016-0402-9. PMID: 27059342.

I AM SURE MY HUSBAND IS BETRAYING ME

"I have come here because I hit my wife."

"You hit your wife?!"

"Yes, Doctor, I have a black eye and my arm still hurts."

"It wasn't my fault, I was sleeping."

"That is the excuse! You have a girlfriend, and you beat me since you no longer can stand me!

"I swear there is no girlfriend. I was trying to protect you, someone was trying to grab your purse in a bus"

"Yes, yes…. he was flying from the bed. It was almost in the morning and I was half-awake. I saw him jump, fall on me and hit me and this is how I am now."

"It wasn't my fault, Doctor, I was sleeping… I mean I was dreaming that I was in a bus and a thief entered and started taking everybody's wallets, specifically yours. It was then that I started fighting him and I woke up with my wife screaming."

"Doctor, in 40 years of marriage he has never touched me, not even with a feather, and now he has hit me twice in the night. The other day I woke up with his hands around my throat. He keeps saying he is dreaming, but I am sure he wants to get ready of me."

"Don't say that, I am dreaming. I am dreaming about fights."

"But I am the one who is suffering, and now I'm afraid. If he doesn't know what he's doing, at some point he is going to really hurt me. 40 years of marriage! He is so calm during the day. I've never seen him quarrelling with anybody, but now I'm afraid. Go to your girlfriend and let me in peace"

This case is very suggestive of RBD[265] *(REM Behaviour Disorder), as explained in chapter 62. Here we explain the consequences upon those sharing the same bed, in this case, the wife.*

Sleeping close to a person with violent behaviours is, in principle, dangerous, why?

— *Both are asleep and therefore less able to defend or to control themselves*
— *The violent behaviours are quite vigorous and therefore potentially quite armful*
— *The aggressor's awakening is not immediate and may take some minutes; this means that he will not stop immediately even one someone is shouting on him*
— *The consequences might be quite dramatic and impact both members of the couple: broken limbs, black eyes, bruised neck, etc*
— *The psychologic consequences upon the co-sleeper must be considered: fear, insecurity and mistrust are possible*

Protection of the co sleeper implies, besides treatment of the aggressor, solutions adapted to each specific case, such as, separate beds or separate rooms

Marital conflicts are evident. Mistrust must be dismissed: there is no guilt is this situation

[265] Dauvilliers Y, Schenck CH, Postuma RB, Iranzo A, Luppi PH, Plazzi G, Montplaisir J, Boeve B. REM sleep behaviour disorder. Nat Rev Dis Primers. 2018 Aug 30;4(1):19. doi: 10.1038/s41572-018-0016-5. PMID: 30166532.

SHE TRIED TO TAKE HER OWN LIFE DURING SLEEP

— Mary - I am quite sad, with no feelings and no wishes. I don't know what to do. I just want to be alone.

— John - We have a small baby, 1 year old, but she does want to take care of him, even after being dismissed from work

— Mary - It is a long history...

— John - Yes, well there were some conflicts with the boss. She complained at the trade union and the whole thing is under analysis. I am quite worried, she was a fantastic mother (we have another son), a fantastic wife and a fantastic worker and som nights ago I saw her trying to take her life while she was asleep.

— Doctor - Trying to take her own life?

— John - Yes, cutting the wrist with a sharp object

— Doctor – Can I speak with her alone for a while?

— John – Yes, certainly

— Doctor – Tell me Mary, what is going on...

— Mary – I had a problem at my work. I was responsible for the logistics of a big supermarket. I had the pregnancy medical leave, and upon my return to work I was not so efficient as before and they changed my position and put me having nothing to do. I complained and they fired me ... I worked there for more than 10 years ...

— Doctor – Is this the only reason why you are so distressed?

— Mary – Well, doctor, my live has always been difficult. As a child my mother was victim of domestic violence since my father was an alcoholic. I helped and supported my mother to get divorced, and when she married again, I have been abused by my stepfather. She did not believe me, and I went to my grandmothers 'home and never spoke with her for many years.

This is probably a sleep-related dissociative disorder associated with a multi traumatic childhood, adolescence and adulthood[266]. In effect, episodes equal to the ones described in the text were recorded during video polysomnography; they occurred during sustained wakefulness.

Psychiatric and psychologic interventions were quite successful in this case.

Trauma, within the family environment, in childhood and adolescence is, unfortunately quite frequent. Consequences persist for life[267].

__Why family hurts their children?__

[266] Eiser AS. Sleep-Related Dissociative Disorders. Sleep Med Clin. 2024 Mar;19(1):159-167. doi: 10.1016/j.jsmc.2023.10.003. Epub 2023 Nov 22. PMID: 38368062.

[267] Paiva, T., & Canas-Simião, H. (2022).Sleep and violence perpetration: A review of biological and environmental substrates. *Journal of Sleep Research*, 00, e13547. https://doi.org/10.1111/jsr.13547

MY WIFE HAS MADE ME SLEEP IN THE LIVING ROOM

My wife has made me sleep in the living room because she can't stand my shouting.

I start shouting and struggle helplessly in a very agitated state. I don't remember anything, but I hurt her because I make these violent movements with my arms.

And that shouting is terrible. She says she's afraid. I don't remember anything. As she can no longer bear this, she has made me go and sleep in the living room and she now sleeps with our daughter with the door locked.

The kid is 3 years old and is sleeping with her mother.

As for me, when this happens, I wake up with my body all smashed up and I get endless headaches.

I'm desperate because you know everything is going wrong. I need to concentrate at work and as I sleep badly so often, I have some difficulties.

My family life is complicated. With her fear, the kid in the middle and my shouting, everything is completely out of control. Our marital life is non-existent, and I feel that things are falling apart.

Shouting when sleeping may have various causes, such as, night terrors, epilepsy, nightmares, panic attacks or functional (psychogenic) crisis.

The described behaviour is probably a sleep hypermotor (hyperkinetic) epilepsy (SHE)[268].

---

[268] Wan H, Wang X, Chen Y, Jiang B, Chen Y, Hu W, Zhang K, Shao X. Sleep-Related Hypermotor Epilepsy: Etiology, Electro-Clinical Features, and Therapeutic Strategies. Nat Sci Sleep. 2021 Nov 13;13:2065-2084. doi: 10.2147/NSS.S330986. PMID: 34803415; PMCID: PMC8598206.

SHE includes sporadic and familial forms, with approximately 86% of cases being sporadic and 14% being familial.

Despite this being another case with violent attitudes during sleep, it is probably a case of frontal lobe epilepsy which can explain the piercing screams, the extensive and strong bilateral limb movements, and the fatigue and headaches in the morning.

This can happen even if there are no seizures during the day, and during the night they are not accompanied by the "typical" signs of epilepsy, namely biting one's tongue and loss of urine.

Be that as may, the diagnosis must be confirmed with a video polysomnography, including 19 EEG electrodes.

The overall prognosis for SHE is unsatisfactory, but different aetiologies affect patients' prognoses

Besides this problem, however, this patient has others which are equally serious: the consequences of all of this to his family life and having a 3-year-old daughter sleeping in her parent's bed.

<u>Shouting during sleep requires clarification of the underlying cause.</u>

MY MOTHER GETS UP IN THE NIGHT AND STARTS COOKING

"Look, my mother won't tell you anything, but I've seen it, I've filmed it. We have played her a recording of it and even then, she says it is nothing."

"It's not quite like that, I know what I am doing, just that I don't think it is important. If I wake up I cook, what's the harm in that?"

"Mum, what's the harm? You've put on so much weight since you started this night time cooking lark. How much have you put on? 15 kg?"

"Well, doctor, I can't sleep and then I get up. I go to the kitchen, and I have to do something. My problem is not sleeping well. I have terrible insomnia, and I jerk, and the starts wake me up.

I sleep just a few hours and after eating I am quieter, and I can sleep a bit more in the morning."

"A bit more, mum? The other day you got up at midday. Whenever have you done that before? And another thing, you have been depressed."

"Of course I have been depressed. I live alone, and you are far way. How do you expect me to feel good?"

"I don't know. What do you think doctor? Is it normal to cook steaks at dawn?"

This case history involves night eating syndrome (NES)[269]. Here, the individual knows that she is awake and is consciously eating.

---

[269] McCuen-Wurst C, Ruggieri M, Allison KC. Disordered eating and obesity: associations between binge-eating disorder, night-eating syndrome, and weight-related comorbidities. Ann N Y Acad Sci. 2018 Jan;1411(1):96-105. doi: 10.1111/nyas.13467. Epub 2017 Oct 16. PMID: 29044551; PMCID: PMC5788730.

Patients don't always cook; some raid the fridge, others prepare supper early, and others leave something to eat on the bedside table.

Patients may wake up once or twice, or even more times. The food chosen is generally full of calories, rich in fats and carbohydrates, and is consumed in an indiscriminate but relatively conscious manner (there may be almost automatic episodes, which the patient may not remember).

The greatest risk is weight gain, which happens due both to the caloric intake and higher nocturnal absorption, due to the nocturnal production of ghrelin, a stomach produced hormone.

Weight gain is generally quite significant and may induce sleep apnoeas. The other risk is insomnia, due to the successive sleep interruptions. Many of these cases are linked to either sleep apnoeas or Periodic Limb Movements and get better with the respective treatment.

Furthermore, NES are also associated with higher risk of psychopathology, including mood disorders and anxiety.

Night eating is often confused with the later food eating habits in southern European countries, and is not considered an abnormal problem but rather, at the most, bizarre behaviour. As such, there are no data for the prevalence of the condition in the general population in such countries.

__Night eating is an illness.__

WHEN I WAKE UP IN THE MORNING THERE ARE CRUMBS IN THE ROOM

My husband told me to come. It's just that at night I get up without really noticing, go to the kitchen and eat whatever is in the fridge. I eat biscuits, bread, fruit or whatever. I have eaten dog food which was being kept in the fridge. You can't imagine how much fun they made of me!

In the morning, I know something happened because I see that look on my husband's face and hear the giggles of my daughter.

They joke with me, and say it is impossible I don't realise what is happening! But I really don't... I have at the most, a vague idea that something has happened.

"Are you fatter?"

"No, I do regular diets, and I am the fatter/thinner type. Sometimes I get the food munchies, even when awake, and eat everything in front of me: everything that is bad for you: chocolates, cakes, sausages, *chorizo*, cheese, and things with loads of calories."

This is sleep-related eating disorder[270]. Patients tend to eat foods full of calories, or sometimes even incredible things: leftovers, animal food, etc., but they do not remember doing this.

What is important is to solve any situations involving stress and investigate if there is a specific food disorder, such as bulimia or anorexia, which is common both in the patients and members of their families.

The treatment is then contextualised within the treatment for this eating disorder.

---

[270] Lipford MC, Auger RR. Sleep-Related Eating Disorder. Sleep Med Clin. 2024 Mar;19(1):55-61. doi: 10.1016/j.jsmc.2023.10.013. Epub 2023 Nov 29. PMID: 38368069.

This can also, as with the previous case, be linked to Periodic Limb Movements, depression or stressful situations. There is often a family history of eating disorders (anorexia, bulimia, etc.).

If you unknowingly eat or drink at night, seek help.

MY SLEEP AND I

I AM AFRAID OF SLEEPING WITH HIM

"I will have to be the one to tell you, as he won't remember anything, but I am terribly afraid.

The other day I woke up and he was grabbing my neck and choking me. I managed to slip away as best I could. Another time I saw him get up, and I went behind him and he gave me a punch in the chest which took all the breath out of me for a while.

But it's not just me, it's also him. Another time he got up and when I called him, he hit his head against the door with so much force that he broke the planes of glass on the door.

I am afraid of what could happen. He is much stronger than me and… I don't know…

I just feel that this is dangerous. I am already afraid of falling asleep. And I lie awake with my eyes open waiting for something. I have always slept well but now I am starting not to be able to sleep."

"At what time does this happen?"

"It's more at the start of the night, around 1 hour after falling asleep. He doesn't remember anything."

"Well, that's not quite so. I have an idea and when I wake up, I'm lucid."

"You're lucid?? The other day you told me you had to go and catch the plane. There was no plane."

"Has something caused this? Excessive physical exercise, or have you been sleeping very little? Or been drinking, worried, feverish?"

"Now that you mention it, I think so. When you grabbed my neck you had fever, when you talked about the plane you had been sleeping very little because you had to do I don't know what."

"And when I gave you that punch, I had taken part in that tennis tournament. Do you remember? It was a week of training and games."

"You will have to do some tests, but from what you have told me, the violence from your sleep is related to confusional arousals or sleepwalking. Did you sleepwalk as a child?"

"Yes, yes, but then it stopped."

"And is there anyone in the family who sleepwalks or something similar?"

"There is, Doctor, my mother-in-law told me that once or twice the same thing happened with his father. But you know I'm afraid, if he comes at me with his hands around my neck."

These episodes of violence linked to sleep are clearly dangerous and should be correctly diagnosed and treated.

In this case, they appear at a certain hour and there is a suggestive series of occurrences point to an increase of deep sleep (exercise, fever, prior sleep deprivation).

Diagnosis is vital and is carried out by video-polysomnography, after having "simulated/provoked" the factors described which set this "on".

Persistence of NREM parasomnias in adulthood, the sleep-related harmful behaviors, non-restorative sleep, daytime sleepiness or diurnal impairment suggest the possibility of a more severe phenotype[271].

---

[271] Mainieri G, Loddo G, Baldelli L, Montini A, Mondini S, Provini F. Violent and Complex Behaviors and Non-Restorative Sleep Are the Main Features of Disorders of Arousal in Adulthood: Real Picture or a More Severe Phenotype? J Clin Med. 2023 Jan 3;12(1):372. doi: 10.3390/jcm12010372. PMID: 36615171; PMCID: PMC9821298.

These cases may have medical and legal consequences and imply objective proof of all the data and facts, should there be serious physical aggression; furthermore, individuals are not conscious of their acts when performing them, but they can be considered responsible for not controlling the factors which trigger the sleep events[272].

__Violence during sleep has various possible causes. Find out what causes it and treat it.__

---

[272] Popat S, Winslade W. While You Were Sleepwalking: Science and Neurobiology of Sleep Disorders & the Enigma of Legal Responsibility of Violence During Parasomnia. Neuroethics. 2015;8(2):203-214. doi: 10.1007/s12152-015-9229-4. Epub 2015 Apr 24. PMID: 26203309; PMCID: PMC4506454.

I HAVE HORRIBLE NIGHTMARES

"I wake up with certain frightening nightmares, which are really unpleasant. It actually hurts to think about them because such bad things happen in them that I am afraid that they will really happen… I have been so tired lately."

"What happens?"

"There are people who die or who have died – unspeakable things – I dreamed that one of my children had died – at other times they are more normal, such as I am falling off a cliff, I can't find the way out or something is doing harm to me.

I wake up in the middle of the night in a bad state and I am not able to get back to sleep."

"What time do you have these nightmares?"

"They happen more in the early morning, around 4:00 am or 5:00 am; I don't sleep anymore."

"Have you been feeling depressed or sad?"

"Well, lately life has not been easy.

My mother died 1 year ago, and I was very close to her. I really miss her. My husband is very distant from me. It's been like that for some time, but now it's worse and I discovered that he has a lover. It was a shock, and I don't know yet what I should do. One of my daughters is sick… Yes, she's sick. She doesn't eat, has anorexia and doesn't eat, and refuses any treatment. My husband can't deal with that very well and gets angry with her. I think his lover is an escape from all these complications and because of that I'm not thinking of separating. We have 3 children… and it would be difficult for them.

My mother was a great help and now that I've lost her, I really miss her. Since she died, I have been looking after my father. Because he is old, he is very stubborn and only does what he wants.

I feel in a rut, everything is going from bad to worse wherever I look. When I was young I was so happy, so full of life."

"Besides this, do you sleep well? Do you fall asleep easily? Do you snore? Do you wake up with a headache?"

"I used to fall asleep quickly, but recently I haven't done so. I toss and turn a lot before sleeping and I think about things, about problems.

The story of my husband has really hurt me. It's a pain here inside which won't go but even so, in a way, I forgive him. Then my daughter is very difficult. We don't know what to do, to complain, to force feed her, to accept it. There are days when I get a knot in my stomach seeing her eat, hesitant between complaining and hugging her. I don't know when everything became so complicated… but the recent years have been so heavy.

You asked me if I snored. No, I don't snore, but these nightmares trouble me at night."

"Do you take any pills, either to help you sleep or for anything else?"

"I take calcium for my bones, and I do substitution therapy. I don't like taking pills very much. My mother was drenched in pills."

Nightmares are frightening REM sleep dreams which result in brusque awakenings in the middle of the night, after which it is difficult to fall back asleep. They are for that reason linked to certain insomnia-type sleep difficulties and provoke or are associated with a certain level of anxiety.

Chronic nightmares develop through the interaction of elevated hyperarousal and impaired fear extinction[273].

Nightmares are more frequent in individuals with more varied personality limits and who are relatively more creative or when there are psychopathological problems.

Pregnant women may have nightmares, often related to the birth of their baby.

Nightmares about negative things, deaths, cliffs, missing trains, labyrinths and roads with no exit are probably due to depression. Major depressive disorder arises as a consequence of several negative existential episodes such as those outlined in the case history.

Despite the patient being depressed, this does not mean that there might not be other illnesses which could, in a certain way, jointly activating the nightmares. Trauma and posttraumatic stress disorder are common causes. Both for men and women, other sleep disorders have to be excluded (apnoea, restless legs and periodic limb movements, etc.), as well as medical illnesses, without forgetting that there are drugs which can cause or aggravate nightmares. The drugs which interfere with neurotransmission mechanisms in the central nervous system have the greatest possibility of provoking nightmares. These include antidepressants, beta-blockers, barbiturates and antiparkinsonian medication, etc. Nightmares may also occur through benzodiazepine, alcohol or barbiturate withdrawal. Treatment in this case would involve suitable treatment for depression, but if there was a sleep

---

[273] Gieselmann A, Ait Aoudia M, Carr M, Germain A, Gorzka R, Holzinger B, Kleim B, Krakow B, Kunze AE, Lancee J, Nadorff MR, Nielsen T, Riemann D, Sandahl H, Schlarb AA, Schmid C, Schredl M, Spoormaker VI, Steil R, van Schagen AM, Wittmann L, Zschoche M, Pietrowsky R. Aetiology and treatment of nightmare disorder: State of the art and future perspectives. J Sleep Res. 2019 Aug;28(4):e12820. doi: 10.1111/jsr.12820. Epub 2019 Jan 29. PMID: 30697860; PMCID: PMC6850667.

pathology or medication involved, these problems would require specific treatment.

<u>Nightmares provoke anxiety.</u>

<u>Nightmares are common in cases of depression, trauma, post-traumatic stress dirsorder.</u>

I AM ASHAMED OF WHAT I AM GOING TO TELL

We've been married for many years. It has always been normal. We married and we had two children, a boy and a girl, and we raised them without any serious problems.

My children are my pride and joy and my reason for living and I am so happy that the first grandchild is on the way.

As you can see everything is OK, but there is this small hurt that is worrying my soul. It's something a bit dark and obscure, and I don't know where to start, or know if it is really a problem, because in every other way I've always been happy.

I'm afraid of being unfair, of seeing problems where they don't exist, and above all I'm ashamed of what I'm going to tell...

He, that is my husband, wants to have sex with me when he is asleep. The problem is not mine, at least I don't think it is, but it's my husband's. Perhaps I am bringing up problems about something normal, but it is very unpleasant, because I don't know if he is here or there.

I'm a bit ashamed to tell you this. We have already had a lot of arguments, and he always denies everything, but that's not true.

I am ashamed, and I don't know how to start, but here goes. In the middle of the night, I wake up and he is on top of me having sex and he continues even when I don't want to. And you know, it just isn't like him. He answers in monosyllables and the next day, when I confront him with things, he denies it, saying that I am making it up. But I'm not, Doctor, I'm sure of what I'm saying, and the worst thing is I don't know what I should do.

These cases of relations or sexual activities during sleep are described as being rare events, but they are probably more

frequent because for many people it's a disquieting topic that they do not like to report or relate.

People do not know the limits between "normal" and "abnormal" and, as a result, they fear they are exaggerating or being unfair.

As in this case, the stories are told in a roundabout manner with frequent hesitations.

The companion often doubts their motives, and he himself has a vague or absent memory of what happened and thinks it improbable what he is told.

There is of course always in these cases the possibility of simulation, that is, the person involved is carrying out a kind of theatre to obtain their wishes, by alleging then not remembering.

The cases related are surrounded in various bizarre events and linked to anomalous situations. The person him/herself may not be aware of what has happened, and the reports come from third parties, most frequently the partner, man or woman.

This phenomenon, designated as sexsomnia.

Sexsomnia, is considered a subtype of confusional arousal, is characterized by recurrent amnestic sexual behaviours, ranging from masturbation to sexual intercourse. The abnormal sexual activity occurs in slow-wave sleep, and predominates in males.[274]

Complex amnestic behaviours frequently occur in the setting of CNS (Central Nervous System) polypharmacy or supratherapeutic doses[274].

---

[274] Irfan M, Schenck CH, Howell MJ. NonREM Disorders of Arousal and Related Parasomnias: an Updated Review. Neurotherapeutics. 2021 Jan;18(1):124-139. doi: 10.1007/s13311-021-01011-y. Epub 2021 Feb 1. PMID: 33527254; PMCID: PMC8116392.

Sexsomnia, is like that of sleep violence and must be diagnosed and dealt with in the same way, being essential to know what is happening, to set up the necessary treatment and to avoid painful or dangerous situations.

Some cases may have legal and medical consequences, and as such it is important to obtain an extremely thorough objective analysis of all the facts, psychiatric and psychological evaluations of those involved, and sleep tests, with video-polysomnography, to attain rigorous conclusions.

Treatment should be set up based on the diagnosis.

There are sexual behaviour disturbances which can occur during sleep.

I HAVE A PROBLEM WHICH IS DIFFICULT TO MENTION

At night I get painful erections.

You know, I can't sleep because of this, because I wake up at night with painful erections.

They are persistent. They wake me at dawn and won't go away.

I am discomforted, troubled, dissatisfied. I've already been to the Urologist.

They spoke about priapism, but it doesn't happen during the day. Just at night.

During the night and during REM or paradoxical sleep, spontaneous erections occur which are not long-lasting. They are more frequent in young individuals and generally lessen with age.

This is a normal phenomenon which does not necessarily have anything to do with erotic dreams because these occur independently of spontaneous erections.

In the case described, the erections, as well as occurring, are prolonged and therefore painful[275]. They occur at daybreak in periods of greater amounts of REM sleep.

They are an abnormal phenomenon due to a cause which is not fully understood, which may be linked to priapism.

Treatment is complex and sometimes not very effective. Antidepressants should be used, since they reduce REM sleep and, therefore, the associated erections. But they may have the secondary effect of the loss of libido or sexual ability, which reduces patient compliance with the treatment.

Painful nocturnal erections are a real problem

---

[275] Wang Y, Zhang J, Li H. Narrative review: pathogenesis, diagnosis, and treatment of sleep-related painful erection. Transl Androl Urol. 2021 Dec;10(12):4422-4430. doi: 10.21037/tau-21-1045. PMID: 35070824; PMCID: PMC8749065.

G. Glossary

The Glossary refers mostly to features of adult sleep, since it is the focus of this book

Other possible reference is:

Sleep Dictionary: Definitions of Common Sleep Terms | Sleep Foundation

Actigraphy – Tracking the body's movement, external light and body temperature over time

Active Sleep – It is an immature form of REM sleep in newborn babies. It is characterized by eye movements, high brain activity, irregular breathing, and an elevated and variable heart rate.

Adenosine – important neuropeptide in energy transfers and when functioning as a neurotransmitter promotes sleep and suppresses arousal; its concentration increases with each hour an organism is awake.

Advanced Sleep Phase Syndrome – It is mainly manifested in an individual's main sleep period, during which sleep onset and wake times usually occur at least 2 hours earlier than the societal norm compared with normal individuals

Anabolic – factor which increases anabolism.

Anabolism – metabolic process which constructs molecules from smaller units. In functional terms anabolism stimulates, for example, the synthesis of proteins and muscle growth and the mineralization of bone. This process requires energy.

APAP – abbreviation for "automatic positive airway pressure". Designates a positive pressure device in which the pressure varies automatically, between a minimum and a maximum, in accordance with the needs of the patient. This pressure is applied to the nose/face/nostrils through a mask and is used to impede apnoeas.

Arousal – physiological and psychological state of being awake. It is mediated by the brain, by the reticular activating system, by the autonomous (or vegetative) nervous system and by the endocrine system. It thus regulates consciousness, attention and information processing.

Atonia – loss of muscular tone, with the muscles becoming flaccid and unable to move.

Awakenings – waking up from any stage of sleep.

Bad sleeper – sleep with either of the following symptoms: increased sleep latency, nocturnal awakenings, fragmentation, short duration, too long duration, difficult morning awakening, non-refreshing, associated with respiratory, movement, behavioural, cardiac, unpleasant dreams or other strange events

Basal ganglia – nuclei which interconnect the brain, the thalamus and the brainstem.

BIPAP – Designates a positive pressure device where the pressure varies during inhalation and exhalation.

Biphasic sleep – Sleep episodes occur twice a day

Bruxism – term used for the gnashing of teeth; the creepy noise has been compared to the noise of witches.

Cataplexy – sudden loss of muscle tone, which can cause the body or parts of the body to collapse, but during which there is no alteration of consciousness.

Caudate – nucleus within the basal ganglia which is important for the control of movement and the learning and memory system.

Cephalalgia – headache.

Circadian rhythm – rhythm which has a period of one day.

Cluster Headache – a neurologic disorder characterized by severe unilateral and recurrent headaches, around the eye, associated with eye watering, nasal congestion, or swelling around the eye on the affected side. Headaches occur in clusters: daily symptoms typically last 15 minutes to 3 hours during weeks or months and free intervals of 1-year or more. Often associated with sleep apnea.

Confusional arousals – is a NREM parasomnia; awakening from NREM sleep is associated with mental confusion.

Cortisol – Cortisol is a corticosteroid hormone from the steroid family, produced by the upper part of the adrenal gland directly involved in the stress response

CPAP – abbreviation for "continuous positive airway pressure". Designates a positive pressure device which, applied in the nose/face/nostrils through a mask, will prevent the collapse of the upper airways, avoiding apnoeas.

Deambulation – the act of walking around.

Delayed Sleep Phase Disorder – It is mainly manifested as a delay in an individual's sleep onset and wake time of 2 hours or more beyond what is considered ideal and compared with a normal individual

Delta waves – also called delta rhythm or delta activity. EEG waves below 4 Hz. By convention, delta waves are considered in sleep when their peak-to-peak amplitude is greater than 75 µV. They are characteristic of Slow Wave Sleep (N3)

Desmopressin – anti-diuretic hormone replacement which reduces the production of urine during sleep.

Diencephalon — region of the brain which include the thalamus, the hypothalamus, the epithalamus, the subthalamus and the pretectum.

Dopamine — Essential neurotransmitter in communication between neurons; It is present in the basal ganglia. Patients with Parkinson's disease are deficient in its production.

Dopaminergic — drug which enhance the action of dopamine.

Dream — Thoughts or images that occur while sleeping. They can occur during any stage of sleep but are most common and vivid in REM sleep.

EEG Sleep stages — The different and characteristic patterns observed in EEG, EOG and EMG during the evolution of sleep along the night; there are 4 sleep stages (N1, N2, N3 and REM) and Wake stage

Electroencephalogram (EEG) — recording of brain activity at the scalp

Electromyogram (EMG) — recording of electrical muscles activity

Electrooculogram (EOG) — recording of eye movements activity

ENT — Ear, Nose and Throat. Also, ORL — otorhinolaryngology.

Enuresis — involuntary emission of urine.

Exploding Head Syndrome — a sensory parasomnia occurring during sleep-wake/wake-sleep transitions and characterized by the sensation of hearing a loud sound, like an explosion.

Ferritin — protein which stores iron inside cells, thus avoiding the toxicity of iron in its free state. There may be low levels of ferritin in anaemia and in restless legs syndrome, and high levels in hemochromatosis and in porphyria.

Fibromyalgia – is a medical is a condition characterized by chronic, widespread musculoskeletal pain, fatigue, cognitive disturbance, psychiatric complaints and multiple somatic symptoms

Ghrelin – peptide produced in the stomach at the end of the day, which increases the absorption of food.

Growth hormone – hormone which stimulates growth and cellular reproduction. It is produced in the anterior lobe of the pituitary gland.

Hallucination – sensation felt as real, such as scenes, noises, sounds, smells or cutaneous sensations, which do not in fact exist.

Health-related quality of life – is a multi-dimensional concept commonly used to examine the impact of health status on quality of life.

HLA – abbreviation for Human Leukocyte Antigen. It consists of a set of antigens residing on chromosome 6. These antigens are essential elements in the regulation of the immune system.

Hobby – An activity people do for pleasure when not working

Hypnagogic – what happens at sleep onset.

Hypnagogic myoclonus – Sudden, brief, involuntary muscle jerks occurring at sleep onset

Hypnopompic – what happens at waking up.

Hypocretin – the same as orexin.

Hypoglossal nerve – It is the XII cranial nerve; it controls tongue movements

Hypothalamus – the area of the brain located below the thalamus which contains the regulatory centres for certain essential functions such as sleep and wakefulness, appetite, circadian cycles, sexual regulation, body temperature, etc.

Idiopathic – term applied to diseases, the cause of which is unknown.

Idiopathic Hypersomnia (IH) – characterized by an increase in the main sleep episode, and by excessive daytime sleepiness; daytime episodes (non-refreshing naps) last 1-2 h and consist of NREM sleep; There is a CNS dysfunction.

Insomnia – difficulty in initiating or maintaining sleep, or have a restorative sleep, when the appropriate opportunities and circumstances to sleep do exist

Jet-lag – the lag between our internal clock and external time, caused by rapid trans meridian travel, such as on a jet plane

K Complexes – normal phenomena of response to stimuli, both internal and external, such as a noise, or a physiological alteration. They have a short duration, less than 2 seconds, and occur in NREM sleep.

Leptin – substance produced by adipocytes (the cells which contain fat) which reduces the appetite. It is part of the system for controlling weight and appetite. Sleep deprivation leads to a reduction in its production.

Light therapy – A treatment for some sleep problems (seasonal depression and circadian disorders) that employs short periods of exposure to a very bright light to alter a person's circadian timing

Lithium – the salts of lithium are used in the treatment of bipolar disease, some forms of migraine and cluster headaches.

Long Sleeper – A person who requires more than 9 or 10 hours of sleep, to feel refreshed and apt for daytime activities

Lorazepam – often used as a hypnotic. It is a benzodiazepine, which is addictive and induces dependence. Brand names include Ativan, Lorazepam intensol.

Mandibular Advance Device (MAD) — The primary purpose of MAD is to move the mandible forwards relative to maxilla in ordered to widen the airway to prevent to closure. It is used in sleep apnea patients and snorers as an alternative to CPAP.

Melatonin — A hormone produced by the pineal gland that helps to regulate circadian rhythm and sleep. Melatonin is normally produced in response to darkness and is blocked by light.

Myoclonus — brief and sudden muscle twitches or jerks.

N1 NREM — sleep phase that occurs at the beginning of sleep, or after alerts from the other phases. It consists of a low-voltage EEG, with mixed frequencies, mainly in the theta and alpha band. It contains vertex waves, and slow eye movements; there are no sleep spindles, neither K complexes nor REMs. In adults it accounts for about 4-5% of the main sleep episode

N2 NREM — sleep phase characterized by the presence of sleep spindles and K-complexes, and by a low-amplitude baseline activity with mixed frequencies. Large-amplitude delta waves are expected to occupy less than 20% of the epoch. It accounts for about 45-55% of the main sleep episode in adults.

N3 NREM — is the deepest stage of sleep, accounting for about 20 to 25% of the sleep cycle in adults. It is characterized by delta brain waves, also known as slow waves, with a frequency lower than 4Hz; the threshold for arousal is high; heart rate, breathing frequency and body temperature decrease.

Nap — a short period of sleep, typically taken during daytime hours as an adjunct to the usual nocturnal sleep period

Narcolepsy — disorder characterized by excessive somnolence, cataplexy, hypnagogic hallucinations and sleep paralysis.

Night eating disorder (NES) – is a form of disordered eating associated with evening hyperphagia (overeating at night) and nocturnal ingestions (waking at night to eat).

Nightmare – A dream with negative content that causes a person to wake up from sleep. Immediately after waking up, a person normally remembers its content; returning to sleep may then be difficult.

Non 24h sleep wake cycle – also known as free-running type sleep disorder. It is the long-term, constant 1–2-h delay in the time to fall asleep and awaken, which cannot be disrupted or affected by a natural and social exogenous 24-h cycle

NREM Sleep – sleep stage in which there are no rapid eye movement. In this stage everything slows down, the electroencephalogram, cardiac and respiratory rate. Movements are possible, but non- intentional.

Obstructive Sleep Apnoea Syndrome (OSAS) – It is a sleep-related breathing disorder with apnea episodes, i.e., complete or partial airway collapse with an associated decrease in oxygen saturation or arousal from sleep. Other symptoms are loud, disruptive snoring, witnessed apneas during sleep, and excessive daytime sleepiness.

Orexin – substance synthesised in the hypothalamus which stimulates the appetite and which functions as a flip-flop switch between sleep and wakefulness.

Oxygen desaturation – reduction in the oxygen saturation in the peripheral blood, which generally accompanies sleep apnoeas. It is measured in absolute values or in terms of the previous value (desaturation in case it is lower).

Parasomnia – strange phenomena and behaviour which occur during sleep.

Periodic limb movements of sleep – sudden repetitive movements of the legs or arms which occur during sleep; the twitches may extend from the legs to the arms.

Phototherapy – treatment with ultra-bright light which imitates sunlight.

Pineal Gland – It is a small endocrine gland, placed in the middle of the brain between the two cerebral hemispheres. It secretes melatonin and therefore plays an important role in circadian regulation. It is a vestigial organ, larger in children and reduced in adolescence; in adults it is often calcified. In animals, it appears to play an important role in sexual development, hibernation, and seasonal mating.

Polyneuropathy – any neurological disorder of the peripheral nerves.

Polyphasic sleep – multiple intervals of sleep and wakefulness throughout the 24-hour day.

Polysomnography – A specialized sleep study that tracks multiple elements including brain waves, muscle activity, eye movements, breathing, oxygen saturation, ECG and heart rate, body position, etc. Polysomnography is typically performed in a sleep clinic or at patients' home and is used to diagnose sleep disorders and sleep characteristics.

Prolactin – hormone produced by the anterior pituitary gland that's responsible for lactation, certain breast tissue development and contributes to hundreds of other bodily processes.

Putamen – structure of the basal ganglia, which, along with the caudate, forms the striatum.

Quiet Sleep – is a form of non-REM sleep in newborn babies (0-3 months); there are no rapid eye movements, and breathing and heart rates are more regular.

REM — Rapid Eye Movement.

REM Behaviour Disorder (RBD) — is a REM sleep parasomnia characterized by dream enactment during sleep, due to loss of the physiologic REM atonia (REM without atonia)

REM Sleep — special stage of sleep during which dreams are more common; it is associated with considerable variation in cardiac and respiratory rate. The eyes move jutting out from one side to another and there is muscular atonia which impedes movement.

Restless legs syndrome (RLS) — a neurologic/sleep condition that causes a strong, urge to move the legs that's at least partially relieved by movement. Symptoms are more common at rest in the evening, prior to sleep.

Restless sleep — Excessive tossing and turning across sleep. It has multiple causes, sleep apnea, restless legs, periodic limb movement, RBD, restless sleep disorder, neurologic or psychiatric disorders

Restless sleep disorder — A recently described syndrome in which restless sleep is prominent and the ferritin level is low. Restlessness is reduced by iron treatment

Reuptake — term used to designate the inclusion of a neurotransmitter in the organelles**.**

Rheumatoid arthritis — Is an autoimmune disorder, resulting in chronic inflammatory disorder that can affect more than just your joints. It can damage a wide variety of body systems, including the skin, eyes, lungs, heart and blood vessels.

Risk behaviours — acts that increase the risk of disease or injury, which can subsequently lead to disability, death, or social problems. The most common high-risk behaviours include violence, alcoholism, tobacco, drug use disorder, risky sexual behaviours, and eating disorders**.**

Screen time – Time spent using electronic devices including mobile phones, tablets, laptops and other computers, and televisions.

Sexsomnia – Sexual behavior during sleep, within the spectrum of parasomnias, occurring predominantly in NREM sleep

Short sleeper – A person who requires less than 6 hours of sleep, in work and free days, without repercussions in daytime activities

Sleep apnoea – breathing pause, which occurs during sleep, in the upper airways, with a duration equal or greater than 10 seconds.

Sleep cycles – period composed of one episode of NREM sleep and the consecutive episode of REM sleep. In the adult there are usually 4 to 6 cycles per night.

Sleep debt – A cumulative effect of an ongoing or extended period of insufficient sleep

Sleep deprivation – not having adequate duration and/or quality of sleep to support decent alertness, performance, and health.

Sleep deprivation – An amount of sleep that is less than recommended based on a person's age and health. While traditionally used to refer only to sleep quantity, sleep deprivation may be used colloquially to refer to insufficient sleep or sleep deficiency.

Sleep disturbance – It has two possible meanings: 1) A disruption in sleep that causes arousal or awakening; 2) A Sleep Disorder.

Sleep duration – is the total amount of sleep obtained, either during the nocturnal sleep episode or across the 24-h period.

Sleep efficiency – is the ratio of total sleep time (TST) to time in bed (TIB) (multiplied by 100 to yield a percentage)

Sleep homeostasis – Sleep regulation process mediated by the sleep homeostat, which aims to maintain a stable balance between sleep and wakefulness, in the environmental framework.

Sleep hygiene — acts and habits that promote the continuity and effectiveness of sleep. They include the regularity of going to bed and getting up, the adequacy between sleep time and individual needs; the restriction of stimulants before bedtime (alcohol, caffeine, etc.), physical exercise, food and environmental conditions suitable for restful sleep.

Sleep Hypermotor Epilepsy (SHE) — is a group of clinical syndromes with heterogeneous etiologies, difficult to diagnose and treat in the early stages due to its diverse clinical manifestations and difficulties in differentiating from non-epileptic events, which seriously affect patients' quality of life and social behavior.

Sleep inertia — The transition period between sleep and wakefulness, during which full alertness is not present

Sleep latency — is the time it takes a person to fall asleep after turning the lights out.

Sleep onset — is the transition from wakefulness into sleep.

Sleep paralysis — inability to speak or move occurring during an awakening. It may be associated with hallucinations, choking or chest pressure

Sleep position — The position taken across sleep; side sleeping (left or right), back sleeping (supine position), stomach sleeping (prone position) or upright (sited or standing). Usually position change.

Sleep Related Bruxism — It is a sleep-related movement disorder with repetitive jaw muscle contraction, associated with tooth-grinding noises.

Sleep related painful erections (SRPE) — A rare parasomnia consisting of nocturnal penile tumescence accompanied by pain that awakens the individual. There are no painful erections awake

Sleep spindles – are normal phenomena in NREM sleep, which function as "sleep gates", that is, when a spindle appears the stimuli which would wake up the cortex are blocked, and in this way our cerebral cortex is relaxed, and we can sleep.

Sleep spindles – EEG sleep micro events, with spindle-like envelope, with a frequency between 11.5-15 Hz, lasting between 0.5-1.5 sec., which arise in a diffuse manner with maximum amplitude in the central leads, and whose amplitude is generally less than 50 µV. They are characteristic of N2 and persist in N3 and do not exist in REM.

Sleep terrors – Also known as night terrors or "pavor nocturnus", are a NREM parasomnia, a disorder of arousal, characterized by episodes of extreme terror and panic associated with intense vocalization and motility, and high levels of autonomic discharge that occur suddenly out of sleep, but the sufferer does not establish communication and is not pacifiable.

Sleeplessness – Persistent inability to sleep

Sleep-related dissociative disorder – Disorder with psychogenic dissociation with mimic of sleep behaviors, mostly parasomnia behaviors

Sleep-related eating disorder (SRED) – Eating while asleep, with little or no memory of eating the next day

Sleepwalking – Also known as somnambulism, is a NREM parasomnia, a disorder of arousal, characterized by walking episodes or other behaviours during Slow Wave Sleep (N3).

Slow Wave Sleep – it is N3 NREM sleep

Sodium oxybate – drug used in the treatment of Narcolepsy, effective for cataplexy, insomnia and excessive somnolence.

Somniloquy – Speaking when asleep.

Testosterone — hormone produced by the male testis that is responsible for development of the male sex organs and masculine characteristics. It is mainly produced during sleep.

Time in Bed — The total amount of time that a person spends in bed regardless of whether or not they are sleeping during that time

Time zone — a zone on the terrestrial globe that is approximately 15° longitude wide and extends from pole to pole and within which a uniform clock time is used.

Total Sleep Period — The amount of time that a person spends from sleep onset to the final awakening

Total Sleep Time — The amount of time that a person spends actually sleeping during a planned sleep episode. TST is the sum of all REM and NREM sleep in a sleep episode.

TSH — thyroid stimulating hormone

Vertex waves — They are like K-Complexes but shorter and with a localisation more limited to the cephalic vertex, i.e., the top of the head.

Wake after Sleep onset — The total amount of wakefulness occurring between sleep onset and final awakening

www.ingramcontent.com/pod-product-compliance
Lightning Source LLC
Chambersburg PA
CBHW032049020426
42335CB00011B/255